The Drug Recognition Guide

The Drug Recognition Guide

Second Edition

Mark Currivan
Wirral University Teaching Hospital NHS Trust
Wirral, United Kingdom

WILEY Blackwell

This edition first published 2021
© 2021 John Wiley & Sons, Ltd

Edition History
Grandios (1e, 2013)

Registered Offices
John Wiley & Sons, Inc., 111 River Street, Hoboken, NJ 07030, USA
John Wiley & Sons Ltd, The Atrium, Southern Gate, Chichester, West Sussex, PO19 8SQ, UK

Editorial Office
9600 Garsington Road, Oxford, OX4 2DQ, UK

For details of our global editorial offices, customer services, and more information about Wiley products visit us at www.wiley.com.

Wiley also publishes its books in a variety of electronic formats and by print-on-demand. Some content that appears in standard print versions of this book may not be available in other formats.

Library of Congress Cataloging-in-Publication Data

Names: Currivan, Mark, author.
Title: The drug recognition guide / Mark Currivan.
Description: Second edition. | Hoboken, New Jersey : Wiley-Blackwell, 2021.
  | Includes bibliographical references and index.
Identifiers: LCCN 2020026490 (print) | LCCN 2020026491 (ebook) | ISBN
  9781119689805 (paperback) | ISBN 9781119689812 (adobe pdf) | ISBN
  9781119689850 (epub)
Subjects: MESH: Pharmaceutical Preparations | Terminology as Topic |
  Handbook | Nurses Instruction
Classification: LCC RM301.12 (print) | LCC RM301.12 (ebook) | NLM QV 39
  | DDC 615.1—dc23
LC record available at https://lccn.loc.gov/2020026490
LC ebook record available at https://lccn.loc.gov/2020026491

Cover Design: Wiley
Cover Image: © Elena Istomina/Shutterstock

Set in 9.25/12.5pt HelveticaNeueLTStd by SPi Global, Chennai, India

C106871-110321

Printed and bound by CPI Group (UK) Ltd, Croydon CR0 4YY

A directory of drug groups based on 10 tutorials that tells students the *who*, *why* and *what* of drug names...
Who is it that gives generic drugs their names;
Why are they given the names that they have;
What those names mean and how to use drug names as a way to identify *what* they are for.

This book is dedicated to all those students who – by asking all the right kind of questions – prompt their mentors into finding all the right kind of answers.

This book is intended for educational purposes only and not as a guide to clinical practice (i.e., prescribing or medication administration procedures).

Contents

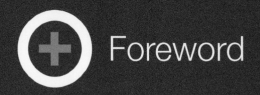

Foreword

This foreword is dedicated to mum.

Welcome to this very creative, special book. This guide to drug classification approaches the topic from a refreshingly new direction. Its innovative use of colour-coding enables the reader to visualise drug names in a way that makes recognising individual drugs and categorising them easier, almost effortless.

Hello, I'm Helen, a registered adult nurse by profession, a former Practice Education Facilitator (PEF) and currently a lecturer in the School of Health Sciences at the University of Liverpool. In my roles both as a PEF and as a university lecturer, I have had the pleasure of working alongside Mark – the author – and we have become trusted friends. Mark is a practice assessor who has written and presented lessons on medicines management that are consistently rated highly by the students. One of Mark's finest qualities is his willingness to listen to the needs of his students, helping them acquire new skills, knowledge and confidence. His dedicated engagement with learners was the catalyst that led to the creation of this book. The care and attention that he has shown in writing the book is remarkable. To outline Mark's commitment, the draft template of the book took nine months to compile – which he did in his own time – whilst working as a nurse and Practice Development Leader on a busy dialysis unit; all this in addition to being a carer to an increasingly frail family member. Delighted to have been asked to write this foreword, I recommend this book to anyone involved in medicines management or anyone keen to learn more about medication.

Helen Potter RGN, BSc (Hon), MEd, FHEA,
Lecturer, School of Health Sciences,
Institute of Clinical Sciences,
University of Liverpool.

Introduction

It is often said that all the really important secrets are ones that are 'hidden in plain sight'. This book is designed to make it easier to learn about medication by showing you how to visually deconstruct drug names in ways that reveal the meanings that can lie concealed within them.

The importance of medication administration as a health intervention is growing. Demographic changes mean that more people are taking increasing numbers of drugs as part of increasingly complex therapeutic regimes (Royal Pharmaceutical Society, 2016). It has never been more important for all those involved in healthcare to have a thorough grounding in the basics of drug classification. Nursing students have long reported that they find medication management one of the most challenging aspects of their training; and many continue to feel that insufficient time is dedicated to pharmacology in the inevitably crowded pre-registration nursing syllabus (King, 2004; Manias, 2009; Dilles et al., 2011; Pearson et al., 2018). This book is unlike other books on pharmacology for students. It emerged from a series of clinical tutorials developed for nursing students working and learning on acute hospital wards – on the 'front line' so to speak. It was devised by a nursing assessor in response to requests from students to help them become more proficient in drug administration; the students having asked for ways to make it easier for them to identify and classify drugs. The students also asked for help with pronouncing some of the more unpronounceable drug names. This is a common but often overlooked concern. Anxiety about feeling foolish due to mispronouncing drug names can often stop students from asking the sort of questions that they should be asking. This book helps with all of these issues.

This book is a directory of drugs, not a formulary; and so it avoids duplicating the functions of the *British National Formulary* (*BNF*) (Joint Formulary Committee, 2019) or similar tomes. Consequently, it does not profess to offer guidance to those who prescribe drugs; neither does it catalogue drug dosages, side effects or interactions. Such information is readily available in a host of other books on pharmacology. This book is different. It was tailor-made in a format chosen by nursing students to meet particular educational needs identified by nursing students. This helped to ensure that the book's focus remains fixed on drug names and its demystifying and drug-classifying aims.

Name stems are the crucial element in drug recognition. Being able to categorise medication on a prescription list – by identifying medicines by the letters used in the stem of their name (i.e., the drug's prefix or suffix) is like finding a key that unlocks all sorts of useful information. Knowing, for example, that only sulfonylureas have generic names beginning with 'gli-' or that only antiviral drugs have generic names ending in '-vir' enables you to instantly recognise glipizide (see Chapter 8) as a drug to treat diabetes and aciclovir (see Chapter 9) as a drug to treat a viral infection… and knowledge, as they say, is empowering. The guide lists more than 700 drugs subdivided into more than 200 drug groups, categorised by class or usage. This book is intended for general guidance only, not as a way to identify every drug in every drug group; nevertheless, it should be invaluable to you while you are getting to know your drugs more thoroughly. So, if drugs and the way they work is still something of a mystery to you, then this little book will give you a head start and help you identify most of the key drugs that you will need to know. We hope that *The Drug Recognition Guide* will make pharmacology make sense to you and so play its part in helping you become a more knowledgeable and safer practitioner.

Drug names: generic/proprietary

Most drugs will have at least three names: a chemical name, a non-proprietary (or generic) name and a proprietary (or brand) name. To prevent confusion to those who prescribe, dispense or administer drugs, the World Health Organisation (WHO) assigns a unique name to each and every medicine known as a recommended International Non-proprietary Name (rINN). Recommended INNs are public property and promote standardisation and uniformity in regard to the identity of generic drugs all around the world.

Note that while a drug will have only one generic name – which will be recognisably similar in most parts of the world (allowing solely for differences in spelling when written in different languages) – this is not the case with proprietary names. A drug's proprietary name is the trademarked brand name given to it by the pharmaceutical company that manufactured the drug. Some older generic medicines that are out of patent may be made by a variety of different drug companies, which means that the same generic drug may have a variety of different brand names. The drug names that appear in this book refer – unless specifically stated otherwise – to generic INNs only.

Comparison of rINNs in English, French, Spanish, Portuguese and Italian

Atenolol (Eng; French; Spanish; Port); atenololo (Ital). Cimetidine (Eng; Fr); cimetidina (Sp; Port; Ital). Diclofenac (Eng; Fr; Ital); diclofenaco (Sp; Port).

Furosemide (Eng; Fr; Ital); furosemida (Sp; Port). Omeprazole (Eng; Fr); omeprazol (Sp; Port; Ital). Penicillin (Eng); pénicilline (Fr); penicilina (Sp; Port). Prednisolone (Eng; Fr); prednisolona (Sp; Port; Ital). Tramadol (Eng; Fr; Sp; Port); tramadolo (Italian).

Drug names and design motifs

Drug companies use design motifs (in advertising, on promotional products and literature and on the drug box itself) in order to highlight the brand name of their particular product and to make the drug's name more distinct and recognisable. The logos and motifs used include emphasising the drug's brand name by using odd combinations of upper and lower-case lettering; some divide the drug's name into segments or use different colours for each letter; some have parts of the name in italics; some use varying typeface styles, etc. The *Drug Recognition Guide* uses similar techniques (specifically, the colour highlighting of drug **prefixes** and **suffixes**) as a graphic device to make the generic drug names in this book as distinctive and memorable as the brand names seen on drug boxes.

Information about the guide

This is a book about drug names. It is about using the letters at the beginning or the end of a generic drug's name as a way to identify what type of drug it is and what it is for. When a new generic drug is being given its name, the WHO promotes the adoption of a 'name stem' (a prefix or suffix) that is the same as those of other drugs in the same drug class (World Health Organisation, 2013). INN stems, therefore, are helpful in revealing the connections between chemically and therapeutically related medicines. For example:

All ACE inhibitors are given names that end with the suffix '-**pril**' (as in **ramipril**, see Chapter 2) and…

All cephalosporin class antibiotics have names beginning with the prefix '**cef**-' (as in **ceftriaxone**, see Chapter 9), etc.

The easiest way to use the *Drug Recognition Guide* is to look in the **Index of Drugs**. This will give you the page (or pages) the drug is on and the pharmaceutical group to which it belongs. Soon you will begin to recognise patterns in the name stems of commonly prescribed drugs.

Many drug groups have name stems that are so distinctive that it is easy to use them as a way to distinguish one class from another. However, endings such as '-**dine**', '-**ide**', '-**mine**', '-**one**' (pronounced 'own'), '-**tine**', '-**zine**' and '-**zole**' are not uncommon in pharmacology and so cannot be used – in isolation – as a way to differentiate between drug groups. Accordingly, the

Drug Recognition Guide recommends that readers take a more exact and all-inclusive look at drug suffixes. For example: instead of just noting the ending '-**zole**', the suffixes '-**prazole**' and '-**rozole**' respectively can be read to distinguish proton pump inhibitors (i.e., **pantoprazole**: see Chapter 1) from aromatase inhibitors (i.e., **letrozole**: see Chapter 10).

In situations where the letters used in the stem of one drug group are similar or, more rarely, the same as the letters used in the stem of another drug group, then a coloured background – as seen here – is used to highlight drugs that have names with similar lettering.

Colour-highlighting a drug's name stem not only aids recognition but also (by appearing to visually segment the name) makes it easier to read – and therefore – easier to pronounce. For example, the antibacterial agent phenoxymethylpenicillin (see Chapter 9) becomes slightly easier to say with its suffix colour highlighted as **phenoxymethylpenicillin**.

References

Dilles, T., Vander Stichele, R., Van Bortel, L. et al. (2011). Nursing students' pharmacological knowledge and calculation skills: ready for practice? *Nurse Education Today*, 31 (5), 499–505.

Joint Formulary Committee (2019). *BNF 78: September 2019–March 2020*. 78th ed. London: BMJ and the Pharmaceutical Press.

King, R.L. (2004). Nurses' perceptions of their pharmacology educational needs. *Journal of Advanced Nursing*, 45 (4), 392–400 [online]. Wiley Online Library. Available from: doi: https://doi.org/10.1046/j.1365-2648.2003.02922.x.

Manias, E. (2009). Pharmacology content in undergraduate nursing programs: is there enough to provide safe and effective care? *International Journal of Nursing Studies*, 46 (1), 1–3.

Pearson, M., Carter, T., McCormick, D. et al. (2018). Pharmacology training in mental health nurse education: justification for an increase in frequency and depth in the UK. *Nurse Education Today*, 62, 36–38.

Royal Pharmaceutical Society (2016). A competency framework for all prescribers. *Royal Pharmaceutical Society* [online], 2. Available from: https://www.rpharms.com/resources/frameworks/prescribers-competency-framework.

World Health Organisation (2013). The use of stems in the selection of International Nonproprietary Names (INN) for pharmaceutical substances. *Stem book 2013* [online]. Available from: https://www.who.int/entity/medicines/services/inn/StemBook_2013_Final.pdf.

1 Drugs that affect the gastrointestinal system

Aminosalicylates
Antimuscarinics
Antispasmodics
Direct-acting smooth muscle relaxants
H2-receptor antagonists
Laxatives
Proton pump inhibitors (PPIs)

Note: antimuscarinics are drugs that can also be used to treat respiratory disorders (see Chapter 4), bradycardia, genitourinary disorders and Parkinson's disease (see Chapter 5) and nausea and vomiting (see Chapter 7).

Aminosalicylates

Aminosalicylates are anti-inflammatory drugs given to treat gastric inflammation associated with conditions such as ulcerative colitis and Crohn's disease. Aminosalicylates are derivatives of salicylic acid: a natural substance originally obtained from willow bark, which has been used as a medicine for thousands of years (Hippocrates had written about the therapeutic properties of willow as far back as 400 B.C.). The Latin term for willow is 'salix', from which is derived the word 'salicylic'. The active ingredient in willow – salicin – metabolises in the body into salicylic acid. In the nineteenth century salicylic acid began to be produced synthetically.

The Drug Recognition Guide, Second Edition. Mark Currivan.
© 2021 John Wiley & Sons Ltd. Published 2021 by John Wiley & Sons Ltd.

In addition to aminosalicylates, **sal**icylic acid is now the basic ingredient in a number of related anti-inflammatory drugs, including aspirin (acetyl**sali**cylic acid: see Chapters 3 and 6). Amino**sal**icylates have generic names that contain the letters '-**sal**-', resulting in names ending in either '-**salazide**' or '-**salazine**':

- **Balsalazide**
- **Mesalazine**
- **Olsalazine**
- **Sulfasalazine**

Despite sharing the same '**sulfa-**' prefix, do not mistake the aminosalicylate **sulfasalazine** for one of the sulfonamide class antibiotics (i.e., **sulfamethoxazole**: see Chapter 9).

Do not mistake the antihypertensive drug **hydralazine** for an aminosalicylate with a name ending in '-**salazine**'. **Hydralazine** is a direct-acting vasodilator of a type known as a '**hyd**razinophth**alazine**'.

Antispasmodics

Antispasmodics are drugs used to bring symptomatic relief from gastrointestinal muscle spasm in patients with conditions such as irritable bowel syndrome (IBS) (Ruepert et al., 2011). The term 'antispasmodic' simply describes what these drugs do (relaxing intestinal smooth muscle) and does not refer to just one type or class of drug. Medicines that have antispasmodic (or 'spasmolytic') properties include antimuscarinics and direct-acting smooth muscle relaxants.

Antimuscarinic antispasmodics

Antimuscarinics work by reducing intestinal motility (see list of other antimuscarinic drugs in Chapter 5).

- **Atropine**
- **Dicycloverine**
- **Hyoscine butylbromide**
- **Propantheline**

Direct-acting smooth muscle relaxants

Direct-acting smooth muscle relaxants are medicines used to help relieve the symptoms of abdominal colic and IBS (Ford et al., 2008).

- **Alverine**
- **Mebeverine**
- **Peppermint oil**

The suffix '**-verine**' is one that can be applied to any drug with smooth muscle relaxing properties (i.e., the antimuscarinic **propiverine** (used to relax smooth muscle in the bladder: see Chapter 5) and the phosphodiesterase inhibitor **papaverine** (see Chapter 8).

H2-receptor antagonists

An amino acid called his**tidine** is a precursor to histamine; with histamine-2 playing an important role in helping stimulate gastric acid secretion. H2-receptor antagonists (the 'H' stands for histamine) are a particular type of antihistamine that works by selectively blocking histamine-2 receptors (also see H1 receptor-blocking 'antihistamines': see Chapter 5).

H2-receptor antagonists reduce gastric acid secretions and so help protect the stomach's mucosal lining from acid erosion (Keshav and Bailey, 2013, pp. 43, 73–75). Cimetidine – the first H2-receptor antagonist – was introduced in 1976 and soon became the first prescription drug in the world to achieve annual sales worth more than one billion dollars, ushering in (for better or worse) the era of 'blockbuster' selling drugs.

H2-receptor antagonists are prescribed to treat gastrointestinal disorders such as gastric or duodenal ulcers, oesophageal reflux and dyspepsia (Puttmann and Roett, 2011). H2-receptor antagonists (often referred to as 'H2 blockers') can be recognised by generic drug names ending with the letters '-**tidine**':

- **Cimetidine**
- **Famotidine**
- **Nizatidine**
- **Ranitidine**

Note a few exceptions: drugs with names ending in '-**tidine**' but which are not H2-receptor antagonists: **azacitidine** (a chemotherapy drug: see Chapter 10) and **hexetidine** (an antiseptic mouth wash).

Laxatives

Laxatives (also known as aperients or purgatives) are given to treat or prevent constipation. There are various types: bulk-forming laxatives (i.e., ispaghula husk and sterculia) that act by increasing faecal mass; osmotic laxatives (i.e., lactulose) that draw water into the bowel; faecal softeners (i.e., docusate sodium and poloxamer '188') that ease rectal straining and stimulant laxatives (i.e., bisacodyl, dantron, senna and sodium picosulfate) that promote peristalsis and bowel motility. **Co-danthramer** (which combines **dantron** with **poloxamer '188'**) and **co-danthrusate** (which combines **dantron** with docusate sodium) are both **co**mpound laxatives (hence their '**co-**' prefix). Prucalopride is a selective 5HT-4 receptor agonist: it promotes bowel motility by enhancing the transmission of serotonin-4 (5HT-4) to 5HT-4 receptors in the colon.

- **Bisacodyl**
- **Co-danthramer**
- **Co-danthrusate**
- **Docusate sodium**
- **Ispaghula husk**
- **Lactulose**
- **Prucalopride**
- **Senna**
- **Sodium picosulfate**
- **Sterculia**

Do not confuse **dantron** (a component of both **co-danthramer** and **co-danthrusate**) with the antiemetic **ondansetron** (see Chapter 7). Similarly, do not mistake the laxative **prucalopride** for a benzamide class antipsychotic (i.e., **amisulpride**, see Chapter 5).

Proton pump inhibitors (PPIs)

The parietal cells in the stomach release a stream of enzymes known as the hydrogen–potassium adenosine triphosphatase enzyme system (commonly called 'the proton pump'). This is the final (and crucial) step in the process of gastric acid secretion. Proton pump inhibitors (PPIs), as their name indicates, are drugs that inhibit the proton pump, thereby reducing gastric acid secretion. PPIs are effective in treating dyspepsia, oesophageal reflux, in preventing or treating peptic ulcers and in helping eradicate *Helicobacter pylori* (Strand et al., 2017). First introduced in the late 1980s, PPIs are now among the most commonly prescribed drugs in the world (Savarino et al., 2017). PPI names end in '-**prazole**'.

- **Esome**prazole
- **Lanso**prazole
- **Ome**prazole
- **Panto**prazole
- **Rabe**prazole

Note an exception: a drug ending in '-**prazole**' that is not a proton pump inhibitor: **aripiprazole** (an atypical antipsychotic drug: see Chapter 5).

Do not mistake PPIs ending in '-**prazole**' for antibiotics ending in '-**nidazole**' (i.e., **metronidazole**) or '-**oxazole**' (i.e., **co-trimoxazole**) (see Chapter 9); or antifungals ending in '-**conazole**' (i.e., **flucona-zole**: Chapter 9) or hormone antagonists ending in '-**rozole**' (i.e., **letrozole**: Chapter 10) [chemically, all of the above are azole derivatives, hence their '-**zole**' suffix].

References

Ford, A.C., Talley, N.J., Spiegel, B.M. et al. (2008). Effect of fibre, antispasmodics and peppermint oil in the treatment of irritable bowel syndrome: systematic review and meta-analysis. *British Medical Journal*, 337, a2313.

Keshav, S. and Bailey, A. (2013). *The gastrointestinal system at a glance*. 2nd ed. Chichester: Wiley Blackwell.

Puttmann, M. and Roett, M.A. (2011). H2 blockers are as effective as PPIs for long-term relief of non-ulcer dyspepsia. *Evidence-Based Practice*, 14 (2), 14.

Ruepert, L., Quartero, A.O., de Wit, N.J. et al. (2011). Bulking agents, antispasmodics and antidepressants for the treatment of irritable bowel syndrome. *Cochrane Database of Systematic Reviews* [online]. Available from: doi: 10.1002/14651858.CD003460.pub3.

Savarino, V., Dulbecco, P., de Bortoli, N. et al. (2017). Appropriate use of proton pump inhibitors (PPIs): need for a reappraisal. *European Journal of Internal Medicine*, 37, 19–24 [online]. Available from: doi: 10.1016/j.ejim.2016.10.007.

Strand, D.S., Kim, D. and Peura, D.A. (2017). 25 years of proton pump inhibitors: a comprehensive review. *Gut and Liver*, 11 (1), 27–37 [online]. Available from: doi: 10.5009/gnl.15502.

Drugs that affect the cardiovascular system

2

Antihypertensives

ACE inhibitors
Alpha-1 adrenoceptor blockers
Angiotensin receptor blockers
Beta-blockers
Calcium channel blockers
Centrally-acting antihypertensives
Diuretics
Endothelin receptor antagonists
Potassium channel activators
Renin inhibitors

Also

Antiarrhythmics
Cardiac glycosides
Neprilysin inhibitors
Nitrates

ACE inhibitors

When blood vessels constrict, blood pressure increases; when blood vessels dilate (relax), blood pressure decreases. A sudden and unexpected fall in blood pressure produces an automatic response: it triggers the body's renin–angiotensin system; a cascade of inter-connected endocrine secretions that results in vasoconstriction and a consequential increase in blood pressure.

The Drug Recognition Guide, Second Edition. Mark Currivan.
© 2021 John Wiley & Sons Ltd. Published 2021 by John Wiley & Sons Ltd.

Angiotensin-converting enzyme (ACE) inhibitors belong to a category of anti-hypertensive drugs known as vasodilators: drugs that reduce blood pressure by making blood vessels dilate. ACE inhibitors work by blocking the action of ACE, thereby inhibiting the conversion of angiotensin-I to angiotensin-II. This interrupts the renin–angiotensin response and causes vasodilation. ACE inhibitors are given to treat hypertension, heart failure and diabetic nephropathy. Evidence suggests they can reduce the likelihood of cardiovascular disease events and have a reno-protective effect, delaying the progress of chronic renal failure (Cai et al., 2018). ACE inhibitors can be recognised by generic names ending in '-**pril**':

- **Capto**pril
- **Enala**pril
- **Fosino**pril
- **Imida**pril
- **Lisino**pril
- **Perindo**pril
- **Quina**pril
- **Rami**pril
- **Trandola**pril

Alpha-1 adrenoceptor blockers

Alpha-1 adrenoceptor blockers (often simply referred to as 'alpha-blockers') are given for two reasons: to treat hypertension or to treat urinary obstruction resulting from benign prostatic hyperplasia (BPH), a benign enlargement of the prostate. Alpha-1 adrenoceptor stimulation causes blood vessels to constrict, narrowing the vessels and so increasing the blood pressure. Alpha-blockers lower blood pressure by blocking these constricting signals to alpha-1 receptors, making the blood vessels relax and dilate. Phenoxybenzamine and phentolamine are alpha-blockers used to treat high blood pressure specifically related to a condition called pheochromocytoma.

Alpha-1 adrenoceptor blockade can also relax smooth muscle around the bladder and prostate and so relieve the symptoms of urinary obstruction caused by BPH. The most commonly used alpha-blockers have generic names ending in '-**zosin**' or '-**sulosin**':

- **Alfu**zosin
- **Doxa**zosin
- **Indoramin**
- **Phenoxybenzamine**

- **Phentolamine**
- **Prazosin**
- **Tamsulosin**
- **Terazosin**

Do not confuse alpha-1 adrenoceptor 'antagonists' with alpha-2 'agonists' (i.e., **clonidine**: see 'Centrally-acting antihypertensives' section).

Angiotensin receptor blockers

Angiotensin receptor blockers (ARBs) (also known as 'angiotensin-II receptor antagonists') are vasodilators: antihypertensive drugs that work by making blood vessels dilate. Like ACE inhibitors and renin inhibitors, angiotensin receptor blockers are another class of drug that works by having an inhibitory effect on the renin–angiotensin system: blocking an automatic response to counteract falling blood pressure. ARBs are used in the treatment of hypertension and heart failure. Research has also highlighted the role that ARBs can play (again like ACE inhibitors) in managing diabetic nephropathy (Jennings et al., 2007). Angiotensin receptor blockers can be identified by names ending in '-**sartan**':

- **Azilsartan**
- **Candesartan**
- **Eprosartan**
- **Irbesartan**
- **Losartan**
- **Olmesartan**
- **Telmisartan**
- **Valsartan**

Note: valsartan can be given on its own or together with the **neprilysin inhibitor** sacubitril (as the combined heart failure drug **sacubitril** with **valsartan**).

Do not mistake ARBs ending in '-**sartan**' for endothelin receptor antagonists (ERAs) ending in '-**entan**' (i.e., **ambrisentan**).

Beta-blockers

Beta-adrenoceptor inhibiting agents (or 'beta-blockers') are drugs that block adrenaline transmission to adrenergic receptors in the heart, the peripheral blood vessels, the bronchi and various other locations around the body. Consequently, beta-blockers can be used to treat a wide variety of medical conditions: tachycardia, cardiac arrhythmia, hypertension, angina, myocardial infarction (MI), anxiety and glaucoma. When adrenaline stimulates adrenoceptors in the heart, it beats more rapidly and with greater force. So the effect of a beta-blocker on the heart is to make it beat more slowly and with less force, reducing both the heart rate and blood pressure. The first beta-blocker – propranolol – was introduced in 1964. Beta-blockers were the most important advance in the medicinal treatment of heart disease for 200 years (i.e., since William Withering's work on digitalis, see cardiac glycosides). Rang (2006, p. 13) notes that beta-blockers represented a breakthrough in drug development and pioneered modern receptor-targeting drug therapy.

The beta-blockers betaxolol, levobunolol and timolol are used in the treatment of glaucoma and work by reducing pressure in the eye. However, because adrenaline dilates the bronchi in the lungs and opens up the airways, beta-blockers tend not to be prescribed for people with asthma or other chronic breathing disorders (in case they unintentionally cause bronchospasm). But the development of 'cardio-selective' beta-blockers (that try to limit adrenaline blockade to the heart alone) means that – if there is no alternative – people with asthma may be able to have a type of beta-blocker therapy that is safer and more appropriate for them should they require it (see list of cardio-selective beta-blockers).

Beta-blockers have names that end in the letters '-**olol**', '-**dilol**' or '-**alol**'. Note: carve**dilol** and labet**alol** have both beta- and **a**lpha-blocking properties (see alpha-blockers). The more 'cardio-selective' beta-blockers include acebutolol, atenolol, bisoprolol, celiprolol, esmolol, metoprolol and nebivolol.

- **Acebutolol**
- **Atenolol**
- **Betaxolol**
- **Bisoprolol**
- **Carvedilol**
- **Celiprolol**
- **Esmolol**
- **Labetalol**
- **Levobunolol**
- **Metoprolol**

- **Nadolol**
- **Nebivolol**
- **Pindolol**
- **Propranolol**
- **Sotalol**
- **Timolol**

Note the key difference between beta-blockers and beta-2 agonists (see Chapter 4): the former (beta-blockers) are adrenaline-inhibiting 'antagonists', whereas the latter (beta-2 agonists) are bronchodilating 'agonists' that mimic the effects of adrenaline stimulation of beta-2 adrenoceptors in the lungs.

Calcium channel blockers

Blood vessels have a thin coating of smooth muscle around their walls (called the tunic media). When these muscles contract, the blood vessels are squeezed and the flow pressure of the blood moving along them is increased. When those same muscles relax, the blood vessels dilate and blood pressure is reduced. Muscular contraction is dependent upon intracellular calcium (the calcium in muscle cells). Calcium channel blockers are drugs that block the inward movement of calcium into vascular smooth muscle cells; this makes the tunic media relax and causes vasodilation (a widening of the blood vessels).

Calcium channel blockers are multipurpose vasodilators. There are three different types:

Class I calcium channel blockers
Class II calcium channel blockers
Class III calcium channel blockers

The vascular smooth muscle-relaxing properties of the three different types of calcium channel blocker make them useful in treating a wide variety of different cardiovascular conditions.

Class I calcium channel blockers
Class I calcium channel blockers (also known as **p**henylalkyl**am**ines) are vaso-**dil**ators prescribed to treat angina, hypertension or irregular heart rhythms (also see 'Antiarrhythmics' section).
- **Verapamil**

Class II calcium channel blockers

Class II calcium channel blockers (**di**hydro**pyridines**) are given to treat hypertension and angina. A major international research project known as the ASCOT trial (Anglo-Scandinavian Cardiac Outcomes Trial) highlighted the key role of the class II calcium channel blocker amlodipine (when given together with the ACE inhibitor perindopril) in helping prevent cardiovascular disease events (Dahlöf et al., 2005). Nimodipine is used in the treatment of subarachnoid haemorrhage. Class II calcium channel blockers have names ending in the suffix '-**dipine**':

- **Amlodipine**
- **Clevidipine**
- **Felodipine**
- **Lacidipine**
- **Lercanidipine**
- **Nicardipine**
- **Nifedipine**
- **Nimodipine**

Class III calcium channel blockers

Class III calcium channel blockers (benzo**thiaze**pines) work by **dil**ating (widening) the blood vessels. **Dil**tiaz**em** (the drug name's prefix coming from its mode of action and its suffix from its chemistry) is given to treat hypertension or to prevent or treat angina.

- **Dil**tiaz**em**

Centrally-acting antihypertensives

Centrally-acting antihypertensives are different from other antihypertensive agents (most of which tend to act peripherally or on specific endocrine systems) and instead work by affecting the impulses that help regulate blood pressure in the brain. Centrally-acting antihypertensives can be put into two subgroups.

Clonidine and methyldopa are **alpha-2 agonists**. They stimulate alpha-2 receptors in the brain, the effect of which is to cause a reduction in vascular resistance and produce a corresponding reduction in blood pressure.

Alpha-2 agonists should not be confused with alpha-1 antagonists (see alpha-blockers), an entirely different group of peripherally-acting antihypertensives.

Moxonidine is an **imidazoline agonist**. It (like clonidine) works by reducing sympathetic nervous activity in the brain. As close relatives chemically and functionally, the imidazoline agonist moxonidine and the alpha-2 agonist clonidine share the same '-**onidine**' name stem:

- **Clonidine**
- **Methyldopa**
- **Moxonidine**

Despite its '-**dopa**' suffix, do not mistake **methyldopa** for a Parkinson's disease drug (i.e., **co-careldopa**, see Chapter 5). **Methyldopa** does have an effect on dopamine (hence its '-**dopa**' name stem), but its (indirect) effect is to inhibit dopamine activity; an effect that is the opposite of dopamine transmission-boosting anti-Parkinson's disease drugs.

Diuretics

Diuretics promote diuresis: they act on the kidneys in ways that make them pass more urine. They are given to treat heart failure, kidney disease and hypertension. Heart failure can cause oedema: the retention of fluid in the lower limbs. By removing this excess fluid, diuretics (drugs often colloquially referred to as 'water tablets') can help relieve the symptoms of heart failure. Some diuretics have antihypertensive properties, and thiazide diuretics and loop diuretics can be used to help in the management of high blood pressure. Diuretics are often among the most commonly prescribed drugs for older people. They can be put into four categories: loop, thiazide, osmotic and the potassium-sparing/aldosterone antagonist groups.

Loop diuretics
In terms of the volume of fluid that they cause to be excreted, loop diuretics are the most potent kind of diuretic; their diuretic action taking place in a part of the nephron of the kidney known as the loop of Henle (hence their name). Loop diuretics are used to treat heart failure, pulmonary oedema, renal failure and hypertension. The antihypertensive properties of loop diuretics is partly related to their hypovolemic effect (reducing the amount of fluid in circulation). They have names ending in '-**semide**' or '-**metanide**':

- **Bumetanide**
- **Furosemide**
- **Torasemide**

Thiazide diuretics

Thiazide diuretics (and 'thiazide-like' diuretics such as metolazone) are given to treat high blood pressure and heart failure. Studies confirm the efficacy of thiazide diuretics in treating hypertension. The antihypertensive properties of thiazides are a result of increased sodium excretion and vasodilation (O'Connell, 2014).

Thiazide diuretics are sometimes given together with other diuretics or anti-hypertensives in one **co**mbined tablet (hence the prefix '**co**-'); for example: **co**-**amilo**zide (which combines the potassium-sparing diuretic **amilo**ride with the thiazide diuretic hydrochlorothia**zide**); or **co**-**tenidone** (which combines the beta-blocker a**ten**olol with the thiazide diuretic chlortal**idone**). The two most commonly seen thiazide drug name stems are '-**thiazide**' and '-**pamide**':

- **Bendroflumethiazide**
- **Chlortalidone**
- **Hydrochlorothiazide**
- **Hydroflumethiazide**
- **Inda**pamide
- **Metolazone**
- **Xi**pamide

Do not mistake the antiarrhythmic drug **disopyramide** or the antiemetic **metoclopramide** (see Chapter 7) for thiazide diuretics with names ending in '-**pamide**'.

Potassium-sparing diuretics and aldosterone antagonists

Because both loop and thiazide diuretics can cause hypokalaemia (abnormally and potentially dangerous low levels of potassium in the blood), an alternative – or additional – diuretic that does not have the same kind of potassium-depleting effect can be prescribed. The potassium-sparing diuretics are not as potent as loop or thiazide diuretics and so tend to be given as adjunct (add-on) therapy to help conserve potassium levels while being given alongside other diuretics.

The aldosterone antagonists spironolactone and eplerenone also have potassium-sparing diuretic properties. Note: potassium supplements should not be given to patients who are also taking any kind of potassium-sparing diuretic.

- **Amiloride**
- **Eplerenone**

- **Spironolactone**
- **Triamterene**

Osmotic diuretics

The osmotic diuretic mannitol is given intravenously to treat cerebral oedema or raised intra-cranial pressure.

- **Mannitol**

Endothelin receptor antagonists

The endothelium is a thin strip of cells that acts as the interior lining of blood vessel walls. Endothelial cells secrete a peptide known as endothelin-1. When endothelin-1 binds to receptors in the endothelium, it causes vasoconstriction: a tightening squeeze of the blood vessels that increases blood pressure.

Endothelin receptor antagonists are antihypertensive agents that work by blocking endothelin-1 receptors. This dilates the blood vessels in the pulmonary circulation and so reduces blood pressure. Endothelin receptor antagonists are prescribed to treat pulmonary arterial hypertension.

Endothelin receptor antagonists have names ending in the letters '-**entan**':

- **Ambrisentan**
- **Bosentan**
- **Macitentan**

Do not mistake ERAs ending in '-**entan**' for ARBs ending in '-**sartan**' (i.e., **irbesartan**). At first glance, ERAs and ARBs have suffixes that appear very similar, but when you look more closely you can see that their name stems are clearly different.

Note: pulmonary arterial hypertension can also be treated with drugs known as phosphodiesterase inhibitors (i.e., **sildenafil**, see Chapter 8) or with the prostaglandin analogue **iloprost** (see prostaglandin analogues, Chapter 8).

Potassium channel activators

Potassium channel activators (sometimes called 'potassium channel openers') are drugs that cause vaso**dil**ation by relaxing vascular smooth muscle. The vaso**dil**ating properties of potassium channel activators are highlighted by names ending in '-**dil**'. Potassium channel activators are prescribed to treat a variety of medical conditions.

Minoxidil is a drug used to treat severe hypertension. Because of its well-documented side effects, it is usually considered the 'antihypertensive of last resort'. Because minoxidil can cause tachycardia and fluid retention, it is normally prescribed along with a beta-blocker and a diuretic. Minoxidil can also cause hypertrichosis (a growth in body hair), making it – from some cultural and aesthetic perspectives (if not strictly medical reasons) – an unsuitable antihypertensive drug for women. However, this particular side effect means that topical solutions of minoxidil can be applied to the scalp as a treatment for androgenetic alopecia (male-pattern baldness).

Nicorandil is a synthetic **nico**tine derivative that works as a potassium channel activator. It helps prevent angina by **dil**ating the coronary blood vessels, thereby improving the oxygenation of the heart.

- **Minoxidil**
- **Nicorandil**

> **Note:** a drug with a name ending in '-**dil**' that is not a potassium channel activator (but which does have vasodilating properties: hence its '-**dil**' suffix): **alprostadil**. **Alprostadil** is a prostaglandin analogue used to treat erectile dysfunction (see Chapter 8).

Renin inhibitors

When blood pressure drops suddenly or sodium levels decline, the body responds automatically: renin (an enzyme secreted by the kidneys) and angiotensinogen (a protein secreted by the liver) are released into the bloodstream. Renin cleaves angiotensinogen into angiotensin I, which is then converted into angiotensin II by the ACE. Angiotensin II is a powerful vasoconstrictor and the end result of this cascade of endocrine secretions (known as the 'renin–angiotensin system') is to produce an increase in blood pressure.

ACE inhibitors and ARBs were the first antihypertensives that work by inhibiting the renin–angiotensin system. ACE inhibitors work by stopping ACE from converting angiotensin I to angiotensin II. ARBs intervene at the next stage in the process: lowering blood pressure by stopping angiotensin II from binding to angiotensin II receptors.

Like ACE inhibitors and ARBs, renin inhibitors are also a type of antihypertensive that works by affecting the renin–angiotensin system. Renin inhibitors work by blocking renin directly: intervening at an earlier stage in the renin–angiotensin enzymatic response than either ACE inhibitors or ARBs (Pantzaris et al., 2017). Renin inhibitors are given to treat renin-dependent hypertension. The **ren**in-targeting mode of action of this medicine is emphasised by a generic name that ends with the suffix '-**ren**':

- **Aliskiren**

Antiarrhythmics

Drugs given to treat irregular heart rhythms can be classified in a variety of ways: by type of arrhythmia (supraventricular, ventricular or both) or by their effect on the electrical activity of myocardial cells: the Singh–Vaughan Williams classification. As the focus on the following pages is on drug categorisation rather than direct clinical application, the latter (Singh–Vaughn Williams) will be used here.

Class I antiarrhythmics

Class I antiarrhythmics work by inhibiting the electrical conduction of sodium ions through the sodium channels in myocardial cells. They exert what is called a 'membrane stabilising' effect.

Lidocaine, flecainide and procainamide (the latter now rarely used) are synthetic analogues of co**cain**e (recognisable as such by names containing the letters '-**cain**-') that work as class I antiarrhythmic agents.

Note that lidocaine also has 'pain numbing' properties – blocking pain signals to the brain – which means that it can be used as a local anaesthetic.

- **Disopyramide**
- **Flecainide**
- **Lidocaine**
- **Procainamide**
- **Propafenone**

 Do not mistake the antiarrhythmic drug **disopyramide** for a thiazide diuretic with a name ending in '-**pamide**' (i.e., inda**pamide**, see thiazide diuretics).

Class II antiarrhythmics

The non-selective **beta-blocker** sotalol is considered the definitive class II antiarrhythmic agent. Sotalol also possesses class III antiarrhythmic properties.

- **Sotalol**

Class III antiarrhythmics

Class III antiarrhythmics work by blocking electrical conduction in the heart's potassium channels. Dronedarone has 'multi-channel' blocking properties.

- **Amiodarone**
- **Dronedarone**

Class IV antiarrhythmics

Class I calcium channel blockers can also be classified as class IV antiarrhythmic agents.

- **Verapamil**

Class V antiarrhythmics

Digoxin (see cardiac glycosides) and adenosine (a purine nucleoside) have been called 'class V antiarrhythmics', a broad categorisation sometimes applied to antiarrhythmic drugs that do not fit neatly into any of the other four groups.

- **Adenosine**
- **Digoxin**

Cardiac glycosides

Cardiac glycosides are given to treat atrial fibrillation, atrial flutter, heart failure and cardiac arrhythmia (also see antiarrhythmics). Failing hearts work inefficiently and, in an effort to compensate, sometimes beat more rapidly and irregularly. Cardiac glycosides improve cardiac output: they increase the force of the heart's contractions, making each beat more productive; thereby helping control the heart's ventricular rate, slowing an excessively rapid heartbeat and helping the heart maintain a normal rhythm.

Digoxin is derived from digitalis. Digitalis is a naturally occurring cardiac glycoside that was first obtained from the leaves of the foxglove plant. Galen had written about the medicinal properties of the foxglove in the second century A.D. and by the medieval era it was being used in herbal remedies as a treatment for 'dropsy' (an old term for congestive heart failure). Digitalis, however, can be toxic and unintentional poisoning was not unknown. It was not until William Withering's *Treatise on the Foxglove* in 1785 that digitalis therapy gradually began to move out of the realms of folk remedy and into the world of objective, quantifiable science. To avoid bradycardia, consider omitting digoxin if the patient's apex heartbeat is less than 60 beats/min. Digoxin is a drug that has what is known as a 'narrow therapeutic window', meaning that there is a comparatively minor difference between a dose that is beneficial and one that is potentially harmful. Measuring the levels of digoxin in the blood is used to monitor therapy and avoid digoxin toxicity. Cardiac glycoside names begin with '**dig-**':

- **Digoxin**

Nitrates

Nitrates dilate the blood vessels and improve the blood supply to cardiac muscle, thereby reducing the heart's workload and improving its oxygenation. They are used to relieve the painful symptoms of angina pectoris. They are also used to relieve ischaemic pain in MI and to help treat left ventricular heart failure. Nitrates can be administered in a variety of ways: as a sublingual metered spray, as a dissolvable sublingual tablet, in an ordinary tablet form or as an intravenous infusion. When given to treat angina, glyceryl trinitrate (GTN) is administered sublingually (under the tongue) so that it can be absorbed quickly through the capillaries and into the bloodstream. GTN is usually effective in relieving angina within a few minutes. If an attack of angina has not abated after two separate doses of GTN or if the chest pain has persisted for more than 10 minutes, the possibility that a MI might be occurring should be considered and the appropriate response should be initiated. GTN can sometimes interact with other vasodilatory medicines that the patient may be taking, so be aware that your patient's blood pressure may drop after GTN administration (Boyle, 2007).

In contrast to fast-acting sublingual GTN, isosorbide mononitrate tablets (slower to take effect, but longer acting) are given in prophylaxis: to prevent angina attacks from occurring or to reduce their frequency or intensity. Isosorbide dinitrate can be used in the treatment of angina or in its prophylaxis. The suffix '-**nitrate**' makes these drugs distinctive:

- **Glyceryl trinitrate (GTN)**
- **Isosorbide dinitrate**
- **Isosorbide mononitrate**

References

Boyle, M.J. (2007). A dramatic drop in blood pressure following prehospital GTN administration. *Emergency Medicine Journal*, 24 (3), 225–226.

Cai, J., Huang, X., Zheng, Z. et al. (2018). Comparative efficacy of individual renin–angiotensin system inhibitors on major renal outcomes in diabetic kidney disease: a network meta-analysis. *Nephrology, Dialysis, Transplantation*, 33 (11), 1968–1976.

Dahlöf, B., Sever, P., Poulter, N., ASCOT Investigators et al. (2005). Prevention of cardiovascular events with an antihypertensive regimen of amlodipine adding perindopril as required versus atenolol adding bendroflumethiazide as required, in the Anglo-Scandinavian Cardiac Outcomes Trial – Blood Pressure Lowering Arm (ASCOT-BPLA): a multicentre randomised control trial. *Lancet*, 366 (9489), 895–906.

Jennings, D.L., Kalus, J.S., Coleman, C.I. et al. (2007). Combination therapy with an ACE inhibitor and an angiotensin receptor blocker for diabetic nephropathy: a meta-analysis. *Diabetes Medicine*, 24 (5), 486–493.

O'Connell, S. (2014). Assessing and managing primary hypertension. *Nursing Times*, 110 (14), 12–14.

Pantzaris, N.D., Karanikolas, E., Tsiotsios, K. et al. (2017). Renin inhibition with aliskiren: a decade of clinical experience. *Journal of Clinical Medicine* [online]. Available from: doi: 10.3390/jcm6060061.

Rang, H.P. (2006). *Drug discovery and development: technology in transition*. Edinburgh: Churchill Livingstone Elsevier.

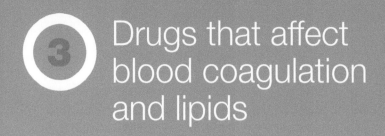

3 Drugs that affect blood coagulation and lipids

Anticoagulants

Direct factor Xa inhibitors
Direct oral anticoagulants (DOACs)
Direct thrombin inhibitors
Heparins
Heparinoids
Hirudins
Prostaglandin analogues
Synthetic pentasaccharides
Vitamin K antagonists

Antiplatelets

Cyclo-oxygenase (COX) inhibitors
Glycoprotein IIB and IIIA inhibitors
P2Y12 platelet receptor inhibitors
Phosphodiesterase inhibitors

Fibrinolytics

Tissue plasminogen activators (tPA)

Lipid-regulating agents

Bile acid sequestrants
Cholesterol absorption inhibitors
Fibrates
MTP inhibitors
PCSK9 inhibitors
Statins (HMG CoA reductase inhibitors)

The Drug Recognition Guide, Second Edition. Mark Currivan.
© 2021 John Wiley & Sons Ltd. Published 2021 by John Wiley & Sons Ltd.

Anticoagulants

A healthy circulation requires that blood has a certain viscosity: blood that is neither under- nor over-coagulated. When the blood is under-coagulated, the risk of bleeding increases. When the blood is over-coagulated, the risk of thrombosis increases. The human body is usually able to maintain a balance between these factors. However, immobility and illness can upset the balance and increase the risk of blood clots. Anticoagulants can reduce that risk. Although often called 'blood thinners', anticoagulants do not, in fact, thin the blood; instead they work by prolonging the time it takes for blood to clot.

Direct factor Xa inhibitors

Direct factor Xa inhibitors are oral anticoagulants given to prevent stroke or to prevent or treat pulmonary or venous thromboembolism. Direct factor Xa inhibitors, together with the oral direct thrombin inhibitor (DTI) dabigatran, are a relatively new group of medicines collectively known as **d**irect **o**ral **a**nti**c**oagulants or '**DOAC**s' (Gee, 2018).

- **Ap**ixaban
- **Ed**oxaban
- **Rivar**oxaban

Direct thrombin inhibitors

Direct thrombin inhibitors are given as an alternative to heparin or warfarin. While dabigatran is given by mouth, argatroban is given intravenously.

- **Argatroban**
- **Dabigatran**

Heparins

Standard (unfractionated) heparin works by binding to antithrombin III (which prevents the conversion of fibrinogen to fibrin) and by neutralising clotting factor Xa (which prevents the conversion of prothrombin to thrombin). This prolongs the clotting time and reduces the risk of venous thromboembolism (Felder et al., 2019). Heparin is given by means of injection. Low-molecular-weight heparin (LMWH) has a longer duration of action compared to standard heparin and is less likely to cause heparin-induced thrombocytopenia (HIT): a reduction in platelet levels that can sometimes occur as an unintended consequence of standard heparin therapy. The LMWHs include dalteparin, enoxaparin and tinzaparin. Heparin names end with the suffix '-**parin**':

- **Dalte**parin
- **Enoxa**parin

- **Heparin**
- **Tinzaparin**

Heparinoids

Heparinoids are a type of glycosaminoglycan derived from heparin (but chemically distinct from it). They are prescribed to prevent deep vein thrombosis (DVT) or as an alternative to heparin for those who are heparin intolerant: i.e., when standard heparin therapy has caused HIT.

- **Danaparoid**

Hirudin analogues

Hirudin is a peptide secreted by leeches that has blood clot-inhibiting properties. Bivalirudin is an analogue of hirudin (i.e., a drug made synthetically to resemble and act like the natural peptide) that works as a direct thrombin inhibitor (see other direct thrombin inhibitors). Synthetic hirudin drug names end in '-**irudin**':

- **Bivalirudin**

Prostaglandin analogues

Epoprostenol is a prostaglandin analogue with anticoagulant properties (see other prostaglandin analogues: Chapter 8). It is used as an alternative to heparin. Epoprostenol is given during haemodialysis to prevent clotting in extracorporeal dialysis lines (Ashley and Dunleavy, 2019, p. 378). Prostaglandin analogues can be identified by the letters '-**prost**-' in their name:

- **Epoprostenol**

Synthetic pentasaccharides

Fondaparinux is a synthetic pentasaccharide (five sugar-based agent). It exerts an anticoagulant effect by inhibiting activated factor Xa. It is given as a subcutaneous or – more rarely – intravenous injection to prevent or treat blood clots in immobile patients or as part of the treatment of myocardial infarction (MI).

- **Fondaparinux**

Vitamin K antagonists

Warfarin was the first and remains the most well-known vitamin K antagonist (VKA). It achieves its anticoagulant effect by interfering with the action of vitamin K (an important natural clotting factor). **Warfarin** was developed as a poison for rats in the 1940s at the University of Wisconsin, hence the prefix '**warf**-' (an acronym of the **W**isconsin **A**lumni **R**esearch **F**oundation). The suffix '-**arin**' is derived from the word '**coumarin**'. Coumarin is a natural anticoagulant found in certain plants that was utilised in the development of the first VKAs. The use of warfarin as an anticoagulant medicine for humans began in the 1950s. Warfarin is used to treat blood clots or prevent them in those deemed to be at high risk (i.e., people with atrial fibrillation, artificial heart valves or rheumatic heart disease). Warfarin therapy requires careful and regular monitoring: a blood test known as international normalised ratio (INR) uses the time it takes for blood to clot as a comparative measure. INR is calculated by comparing the warfarin patient's clotting time with the average normal clotting time. The result is expressed as a ratio and is used to adjust the warfarin dose to maintain a patient-specific target INR value above average normal levels. An INR below target may require an increase in the warfarin dose; if above target, dose reduction is likely. Note: a high INR (5.0 or above) may indicate over-anticoagulation, and it means that there is an increased risk of bleeding.

- **Acenocoumarol**
- **Phenindione**
- **Warfarin**

Antiplatelets

Antiplatelet drugs exert their protective effects by inhibiting platelet adhesion and aggregation. There are four distinct classes.

Cyclo-oxygenase (COX) inhibitors
Aspirin (acetylsalicylic acid) inhibits the enzyme cyclo-oxygenase (COX). Inhibiting COX enzymes affects both prostaglandin and thromboxane. Prostaglandin is involved in transmitting pain impulses to the brain (hence aspirin's analgesic effect: see Chapter 6). Thromboxane helps bind platelets together as part of the clotting process (hence the word 'thrombosis' and aspirin's antiplatelet effect). Since it was first introduced in 1899, aspirin has remained one of the most commonly used drugs in the world. First used as a painkiller, aspirin is now more often prescribed to prevent or treat cardiovascular disease or stroke.

- **As**pirin

Glycoprotein IIb and IIIa inhibitors
Glycoproteins play a role in blood coagulation. Glycoprotein IIb and IIIa inhibitors are drugs that work by stopping **fib**rinogen from binding to glycoprotein

IIb and glycoprotein IIIa receptors on platelet cells. This inhibits platelet cluster-ing and the formation of blood clots. Glycoprotein IIb and IIIa inhibitors are given by means of intravenous injection or infusion.

- **Eptifibatide**
- **Tirofiban**

P2Y12 platelet receptor antagonists
Drugs that block P2Y12 receptors on platelet cells interfere with platelet aggregation and, by so doing, act as 'antithrombotic agents' (drugs given to prevent blood clots). Their use can reduce the risk of stroke and other cardio-vascular disease events.

- **Cangrelor**
- **Clopidogrel**
- **Prasugrel**
- **Ticagrelor**

Phosphodiesterase inhibitors
Dipyridamole is given to prevent thrombosis or stroke. The antiplatelet action of dipyridamole is complex and multifaceted. Dipyridamole inhibits an enzyme called phosphodiesterase (see other phosphodiesterase inhibitors: Chapter 8). Rarely given as monotherapy (on its own), dipyridamole is more often given along with other antiplatelet agents (most frequently, aspirin). Dipyridamole gets its name from **pyri**mi**d**o-**pyri**midine, the chemical compound from which it was originally derived. Anagrelide is a phosphodiesterase type-3 inhibitor that inter-feres with platelet production in the bone marrow. Although originally developed as an antithrombotic agent, the use of anagrelide is now reserved to treat throm-bocythaemia, a disorder that results in increased platelet production.

- **Anagrelide**
- **Dipyridamole**

Fibrinolytics

A substance in the blood called fibrin plays a key role in the clotting process by helping to form thrombi. While the clotting process is an essential element in maintaining haemostasis, any dislodged blood clots loose in the circulation can be very dangerous.

Fibrinolytics are thrombolytic agents: medicines colloquially referred to as 'clot busters'. Fibrinolytics work in ways that differ from anticoagulants and antiplatelets, and instead work by activating plasminogen to form plasmin. Plasmin has a degrading effect on fibrin, and so these drugs exert fibrinolytic properties (breaking up and dissolving blood clots).

Fibrinolytics are given to treat MI and acute ischaemic stroke. Urokinase and alteplase are sometimes also used to help restore patency to occluded central venous catheters (Davies et al., 2004). Alteplase, reteplase and tenecteplase are fibrinolytics of a type known as **tissue plasminogen activators or tPA**. Close monitoring is required when a fibrinolytic drug is administered because it can increase the risk of haemorrhage.

Note: the fibrinolytic drug **strepto**kinase was derived from the bacteria **strepto**cocci, hence its recognisable prefix. Fibrinolytics can be identified by generic names ending in '-**kinase**' or '-**teplase**':

- Alteplase
- Reteplase
- Streptokinase
- Tenecteplase
- Urokinase

Lipid-regulating agents

Cholesterol and triglycerides are lipids present in the blood. Elevated levels of particular lipids in the blood are considered to increase the risk of cardiovascular disease and stroke. Drugs that lower elevated blood lipid levels are known as 'hypolipidaemic' or 'lipid-regulating' agents and they include:

Bile acid sequestrants
Cholesterol absorption inhibitors
Fibrates
Miscellaneous lipid-regulating agents
MTP inhibitors
PCSK9 inhibitors
Statins (HMG CoA reductase inhibitors)

Bile acid sequestrants
Bile acid sequestrants are drugs that bind to bile acids in the gastrointestinal system. This prevents bile acid from being reabsorbed and promotes its excretion from the body. When bile acid is excreted, the liver responds by converting cholesterol into bile acid in an effort to restore bile acid levels – the effect of which is to reduce the levels of **choles**terol in the blood. Bile acid sequestrant names begin with the prefix '**coles-**':

- **Coles**evelam
- **Coles**tipol
- **Coles**tyramine

Be aware of a drug beginning with '**cole**-' (but not '**coles**-') that is not a bile acid sequestrant: **colecalciferol** (a vitamin D3 supplement).

Cholesterol absorption inhibitors

Ezetimibe lowers cholesterol levels by reducing the absorption of cholesterol in the intestines. Research indicates that combination therapy involving ezetimibe and a statin (see statins) can sometimes be more effective than either drug given alone (NICE, 2016).

- **Ezetimibe**

Fibrates

Fibrates (or 'clofibrate derivatives') are drugs derived from **fib**ric acid. Their effect is to cause a reduction in triglyceride levels and an increase in HDL cholesterol ('good cholesterol') levels. Fibrates have names that end in the suffixes '-**fibrate**' or '-**fibrozil**':

- **Beza**fibrate
- **Cipro**fibrate
- **Feno**fibrate
- **Gem**fibrozil

Miscellaneous lipid-regulating agents

Cholesterol lowering medicines are many and varied and include nicotinic acid (and derivatives of nicotinic acid such as acipimox) and the omega-3 fatty acids, the latter being derived from fish oils.

- **Acipimox**
- **Nico**tinic acid
- **Omega-3 acid ethyl esters**

MTP inhibitors

The **mi**crosomal **t**riglyce**ri**de transfer **p**rotein (known by the acronym MTP) is involved in the process by which very low-density lipoproteins (VLDL) are produced in the liver. MTP inhibitors are a class of cholesterol-lowering medicine that works by blocking MTP, thereby reducing VLDL production and lowering blood cholesterol levels. Lomitapide is used to treat a particularly severe kind of familial hyperlipidaemia.

- **Lomitapide**

PCSK9 inhibitors

Proprotein convertase subtilisin/kexin type 9 (PCSK9) is an enzyme involved in lipid regulation and synthesis. Inhibiting the PCSK9 enzyme can help lower elevated cholesterol levels. PCSK9 inhibitors are a relatively new group of lipid-lowering medicines that are used to treat severe hyperlipidaemia or hyperlipidaemia that has failed to respond to more conventional lipid-lowering medicines. They are given by means of subcutaneous injection. PCSK9 inhibitors are a type of synthetic antibody known as **m**onoclonal **anti**bodies (see other monoclonal antibodies in Chapters 4 and 10). Monoclonal antibodies work by binding to targeted cells. The PCSK9-inhibiting monoclonal antibodies specifically target PCSK9, blocking its action and so helping lower cholesterol levels.

- **Alirocumab**
- **Evolocumab**

Statins (HMG CoA reductase inhibitors)

3-Hydroxy-3-methylglutaryl coenzyme A (HMG CoA) reductase inhibitors (drugs now almost universally referred to as 'statins') are the most well-known, well-researched and widely used hypolipidaemic (lipid-lowering) agents. Statins work by reducing cholesterol production in the liver.

The evidence that statin therapy can reduce the risk of cardiovascular disease events has accumulated over the years (Ford, 2013; Collins et al., 2016). Statins are perhaps the definitive example of a drug group that have become known by the letters at the end of their name: the suffix '-statin' not only makes these drugs recognisable but has also become the accepted term for all drugs in this class. Statins, to be strictly accurate, have names ending with the letters '-**vastatin**':

- **Atorvastatin**
- **Fluvastatin**
- **Pravastatin**
- **Rosuvastatin**
- **Simvastatin**

Note three drugs with the suffix '-**statin**' (but not '-**vastatin**') that are not cholesterol-lowering agents:

Cilastatin: an enzyme inhibitor given together with the carbapenem antibiotic **imipenem** (see Chapter 9).

Nystatin: an antifungal drug (see Chapter 9).

Pentostatin: a chemotherapy drug (see Chapter 10).

References

Ashley, C. and Dunleavy, A. (2019). *The renal drug handbook*. 5th ed. Boca Raton: CRC Press.

Collins, R., Reith, C., Emberson, J., et al. (2016). Interpretation of the evidence for the efficacy and safety of statin therapy. *Lancet*, 388 (10059), 2532–2561.

Davies, J., Casey, J., Li, C., et al. (2004). Restoration of flow following haemodialysis catheter thrombus: analysis of rt-PA infusion in tunnelled dialysis catheters. *Journal of Clinical Pharmacy and Therapeutics*, 29 (6), 517–520.

Felder, S., Rasmussen, M.S., King, R., et al. (2019). Prolonged thromboprophylaxis with low molecular weight heparin for abdominal or pelvic surgery. *Cochrane Database of Systematic Reviews* [online]. Available from: doi: 10.1002/14651858.CD004318.pub4.

Ford, H. (2013). The use of statins to reduce the risk of cardiovascular disease in adults. *Nursing Standard*, 27 (39), 48–56.

Gee, E. (2018). Principles and nursing management of anticoagulation. *Nursing Standard*, 32 (23), 50–63.

NICE [National Institute for Health and Care Excellence] (2016). Ezetimibe for treating primary heterozygous-familial and non-familial hypercholesterolaemia. *Technology Appraisal Guidance (TA385)* [online]. Available from: https://www.nice.org.uk/guidance/ta385/chapter/3-Evidence.

Drugs that affect the respiratory system

Antimuscarinics
Beta-2 agonists
Corticosteroids
Leukotriene receptor antagonists
Monoclonal antibodies
Phosphodiesterase type-4 inhibitors
Xanthines

Note: antimuscarinics are drugs that are also used to treat gastro-intestinal disorders (see Chapter 1), bradycardia, genitourinary disorders and Parkinson's disease (see Chapter 5) and nausea (see Chapter 7).

Respiratory disease drugs

Respiratory disease drugs are given to relieve shortness of breath and treat conditions such as asthma, bronchitis, emphysema and chronic obstructive pulmonary disease (COPD). These drugs increase lung capacity either by reducing inflammation or by causing bronchodilation (dilating the airway). The term 'bronchodilator' is, of course, a description of a mechanism of action and does not refer to just one particular class or type of medicine. The medication given to treat respiratory disorders include:

Antimuscarinics
Beta-2 agonists

The Drug Recognition Guide, Second Edition. Mark Currivan.
© 2021 John Wiley & Sons Ltd. Published 2021 by John Wiley & Sons Ltd.

Corticosteroids
Leukotriene receptor antagonists
Monoclonal antibodies
Phosphodiesterase (PDE) type-4 inhibitors
Xanthines

Antimuscarinics

Moulton and Fryer (2011) state that antimuscarinics make highly effective bronchodilators. They work by selectively blocking the broncho-constricting and mucus-secreting action of acetylcholine, stopping it from binding to muscarinic receptors. This relaxes smooth muscle in the airway and reduces secretions (see list of other antimuscarinics in Chapter 5).

- **Aclidinium**
- **Glycopyrronium**
- **Ipratropium**
- **Tiotropium**
- **Umeclidinium**

Beta-2 agonists

Beta-2 agonists stimulate beta-2 adrenergic receptors in the lungs, relaxing respiratory smooth muscle and causing bronchodilation (note the important distinction between **beta-2 agonists** and **beta-blockers**: see beta-blocker summary). Beta-2 agonists can be put into two groups: short-acting (salbutamol and terbutaline) and long-acting (bambuterol, formoterol, indacaterol, olodaterol, salmeterol and vilanterol). The short-acting beta-2 agonist salbutamol has become a mainstay of asthma management; while the longer-acting beta-2 agonists are increasingly being given with other medicines in one combination inhaler (Di Marco et al., 2017; Oba et al., 2018): for example, formoterol with the antimuscarinic aclidinium or salmeterol with the corticosteroid fluticasone. Beta-2 agonists can be recognised by names ending in '-(**bu**)**terol**', '-**butaline**' or '-**butamol**':

- **Bambuterol**
- **Formoterol**
- **Indacaterol**
- **Olodaterol**
- **Salbutamol**
- **Salmeterol**

- **Terbutaline**
- **Vilanterol**

 Do not mistake **ethambutol** (an antimycobacterial agent used in the treatment of tuberculosis) for a beta-2 agonist with a name ending in '**-buterol**'.

Corticosteroids

Inhaled corticosteroids are used to relieve shortness of breath and work by reducing inflammation and swelling locally in the airways (Daley-Yates, 2015). Commonly administered via an inhaler, 'steroids' are often given together with other medicines in combination inhalers (see beta-2 agonists). During acute exacerbations of asthma, a short course of treatment with corticosteroid tablets (usually **prednisolone**) may be necessary (Burns, 2013) (see other corticosteroids: Chapter 8). The inhaled steroidal respiratory drugs have generic names ending in '-**metasone**', '-**sone**' or '-**sonide**':

- **Beclometasone**
- **Budesonide**
- **Ciclesonide**
- **Fluticasone**
- **Mometasone**

Leukotriene receptor antagonists

Leukotriene receptor antagonists are drugs that reduce inflammation in the airway by stopping inflammatory mediators known as leukotrienes from binding to leukotriene receptors (Migoya et al., 2004; Liu et al., 2015). The name monte**luk**ast is informative: it tells you both how the drug works (by means of **leuk**otriene inhibition) and what it is for (the suffix '-**ast**' coming from the prefix in the word **ast**hma, indicating a drug with anti-**ast**hmatic and anti-inflammatory properties).

- **Montelukast**

Monoclonal antibodies

These drugs are synthetic antibodies given by subcutaneous injection or intravenous infusion. They are prescribed to treat severe eosinophilic asthma (see other monoclonal antibodies in Chapters 3 and 10).

- **Benralizumab**
- **Mepolizumab**

- **Omalizumab**
- **Reslizumab**

Phosphodiesterase type-4 inhibitors

Phosphodiesterase (PDE) is an enzyme. Inhibiting the type-4 PDE enzyme reduces inflammation in the airway (see other PDE inhibitors: Chapter 8). The '-**ast**' suffix (see leukotriene receptor antagonists section) seen in the name roflumil**ast** highlights its anti-inflammatory properties.

- **Roflumilast**

Xanthines

Xanthines work by relaxing respiratory smooth muscle and may also have some anti-inflammatory effect.

- **Aminophylline**
- **Theophylline**

> **Note:** the peripheral vasodilator **pentoxifylline** (used to treat peripheral vascular disease) is a xanthine derivative, which explains its '-**fylline**' name stem.

References

Burns, D. (2013). Managing acute asthma in primary care. *Nursing Times*, 109 (42), 17–20.

Daley-Yates, P.T. (2015). Inhaled corticosteroids: potency, dose equivalence and therapeutic index. *British Journal of Clinical Pharmacology*, 80 (3), 372–380.

Di Marco, F., Santus, P., Scichilone, N. et al. (2017). Symptom variability and control in COPD: advantages of dual bronchodilation therapy. *Respiratory Medicine*, 125, 49–56.

Liu, F., Ouyang, J., Sharma, A.N. et al. (2015). Leukotriene inhibitors for bronchiolitis in infants and young children. *Cochrane Database of Systematic Reviews* [online]. Available from: doi:10.1002/14651858.CD010636.pub2.

Migoya, E., Kearns, G.L., Hartford, A. et al. (2004). Pharmacokinetics of montelukast in asthmatic patients 6 to 24 months old. *Journal of Clinical Pharmacology*, 44 (5), 487–494 [online]. Wiley Online Library. Available from: doi: 10.1177/0091270004264970.

Moulton, B.C. and Fryer, A.D. (2011). Muscarinic receptor antagonists, from folklore to pharmacology; finding drugs that actually work in asthma and COPD. *British Journal of Pharmacology*, 163 (1), 44–52.

Oba, Y., Keeney, E., Ghatehorde, N. et al. (2018). Dual combination therapy versus long-acting bronchodilators alone for COPD: a systematic review and network meta-analysis. *Cochrane Database of Systematic Reviews* [online]. Available from: doi: 10.1002/14651858.CD012620.pub2.

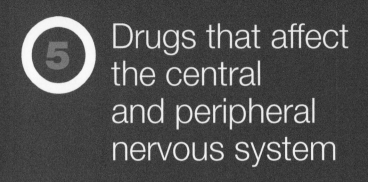

5 Drugs that affect the central and peripheral nervous system

Antiepileptic drugs
Antidepressants
Antipsychotics
Benzodiazepines
Non-benzodiazepine hypnotics
Melatonin receptor agonists
Antihistamines
Antimuscarinics
Parkinson's disease drugs

 Note: antimuscarinics are drugs that can also be used to treat gastrointestinal disorders (see Chapter 1), respiratory disorders (see Chapter 4) and nausea and vomiting (see Chapter 7).

 Note: analgesics also affect the central nervous system. However, due to their specialised role, they have been listed separately in Chapter 6.

Antiepileptic drugs

Antiepileptic drugs (or AEDs) are drugs that prevent or treat epileptic seizures. Epileptic seizures are the result of a surge in electrical activity in the brain.

The Drug Recognition Guide, Second Edition. Mark Currivan.
© 2021 John Wiley & Sons Ltd. Published 2021 by John Wiley & Sons Ltd.

The aim of AED therapy is to restrain the flood of neurochemical signals that result in a seizure. The term 'antiepileptic' (sometimes called 'anticonvulsant') is a broad label that can be applied to any drug – and there are many different types – used in the management of epilepsy. The first effective AEDs were the **barb**iturates (i.e., pheno**barb**ital). However, they have since been joined by an expanding array of newer AEDs: hydantoins, dibenzazepines, benzodiazepines, GABA reuptake inhibitors, GABA analogues, racetam derivatives and many more (Rossetti, 2016). Below is a list of the benzodiazepines used in the treatment of epilepsy (also see separate section 'Benzodiazepines'):

- **Clob**azam
- **Clon**azepam
- **Di**azepam
- **Lor**azepam
- **Mid**azolam

Many antiepileptics (including the benzodiazepines) work by affecting the neurotransmitter gamma-aminobutyric acid (GABA): a neurotransmitter that decreases neuronal excitability, thereby helping keep epileptic symptoms under control. AED therapy may involve just one drug (monotherapy) or two or more different AEDs (polytherapy). The choice of AED may depend upon the type of seizure, drug interactions or the gender – and childbearing age – of the patient. See following list of most (but not all) of the non-benzodiazepine AEDs in current use:

Note: carbamazepine, gabapentin and pregabalin are also used to treat neuralgia (nerve pain). The variety of types can make identifying AEDs by their name stem complex: however, GABA reuptake inhibitor and GABA analogue names often contain '-**gab**-' or '-**gaba**-'; hydan**toin** names end in '-**ytoin**'; **racetam** derivatives have the suffix '-**racetam**'; per**ampa**nel is an **AMPA** receptor antagonist; while dibenz**azepine** names often include the letters '-**carb**-' and '-**azepine**':

- **Briva**racetam
- **Carbam**azepine
- **Eslicarb**azepine
- **Ethosuximide**
- **Fosphenytoin**
- **Gaba**pentin
- **Lacosamide**
- **Lamotrigine**
- **Levetiracetam**

- Oxcarbazepine
- Perampanel
- Phenobarbital
- Phenytoin
- Pregabalin
- Primidone
- Sodium valproate
- Tiagabine
- Topiramate
- Vigabatrin
- Zonisamide

Antidepressants

Antidepressants are drugs given to alleviate depressive mood disorders. Depression is a common condition that often goes unrecognised and untreated (Esiwe et al., 2016). Untreated (or under-treated) depression can have a detrimental impact on health outcomes. Most antidepressants work by prolonging the action of specific neurotransmitters in the brain, serotonin and noradrenaline in particular.

Monoamine oxidase inhibitors (MAOIs)

Monoamine oxidase (MAO) are enzymes found in nerve fibres that inactivate neurotransmitters. Monoamine oxidase inhibitors (MAOIs) are drugs that block MAO, the effect of which is to prevent the inactivation and breakdown of serotonin and noradrenaline, thereby prolonging their action and beneficial effects. Unlike other MAOI antidepressants (that have an irreversible effect on MAO), moclobemide is a 'reversible inhibitor of monoamine oxidase type A', and so is sometimes classified under the acronym RIMA.

- Isocarboxazid
- Moclobemide
- Phenelzine
- Tranylcypromine

Note a sub-group among the MAOIs: drugs called monoamine oxidase-B inhibitors (see Parkinson's disease drugs). The MAO-B inhibitors selectively block the inactivation and breakdown of dopamine, making them useful drugs in treating Parkinson's disease.

Serotonin and/or noradrenaline reuptake inhibitors (SSRI, NRI, SNRI and SMS)

Although it has proved difficult to definitively establish a direct link, it is widely accepted that there is an association between a predisposition to depression and low levels of serotonin and noradrenaline activity in the brain. Serotonin and/or noradrenaline reuptake inhibitors (NRIs) are drugs that selectively inhibit the biochemical recycling of these neurotransmitters, thereby prolonging their action and purported mood-lifting and anxiety-reducing effects. Most of the antidepressants listed below are selective **ser**otonin reuptake inhibitors (SSRIs). However, reboxetine is a NRI; duloxetine and venlafaxine are both **ser**otonin and noradrenaline reuptake inhibitors (SNRIs); while vortioxetine can be classified as a **ser**otonin modulator and stimulator (SMS). Note that the SNRI duloxetine has certain antimuscarinic properties that means it can also be used to treat urinary incontinence.

- **Citalopram**
- **Duloxetine**
- **Escitalopram**
- **Fluoxetine**
- **Fluvoxamine**
- **Paroxetine**
- **Reboxetine**
- **Sertraline**
- **Venlafaxine**
- **Vortioxetine**

Tricyclic antidepressants (TCAs)

Tricyclic antidepressants (TCAs) enhance noradrenaline and serotonin transmission. The chemical name for serotonin is 5-hydroxytryptamine, often abbreviated to 5-HT. In addition to their role in treating depression, TCAs can also be used to help combat a variety of other disorders: neuropathic pain, obsessive–compulsive disorder, panic disorder and eczema-associated pruritus. TCAs sometimes cause unwelcome side effects: drowsiness, heart block, cardiac arrhythmia and various antimuscarinic effects (constipation, urinary retention, dry mouth, etc.). However, the sedating effect of some TCAs may be of benefit to depressed patients who are also anxious or agitated. Tricyclic antidepressant drug name stems ('-**epin**', '-**pramine**' and '-**triptyline**') are derived from letters found in the word noradren**aline** and the full chemical name for serotonin (5-hydroxy**tryptamine**):

- **Amitriptyline**
- **Clomipramine**

- Dosulepin
- Doxepin
- Imipramine
- Lofepramine
- Nortriptyline
- Trimipramine

Note an exception: despite its 'tript-' prefix, do not mistake the sex hormone antagonist **triptorelin** (see Chapter 10) for a serotonin-affecting antidepressant.

Miscellaneous antidepressants

The miscellaneous antidepressants include all those that cannot be put neatly into any of the main antidepressant drug groups (the MAOIs, SSRIs and TCAs, etc.). Ago**melat**ine is a **melat**onin-receptor agonist used in the treatment of severe depressive episodes. The serotonin receptor agonist buspirone is given for its 'anxiolytic' (anxiety-reducing) properties. Lithium is a mood stabiliser given to treat bipolar disorder (manic depression). Mian**ser**in (its '-**ser**-' infix highlighting its effect on **ser**otonin) and mirtazapine are often referred to as 'tricyclic-related' or 'tetracyclic' antidepressants (mirtazapine being a derivative of mianserin). **Traz**odone is a **triaz**olopyridine: a serotonin uptake inhibitor that has anxiolytic properties as well as those of an antidepressant. **Trypt**ophan is a precursor of serotonin (5-hydroxy**trypt**amine). Note: some antipsychotic drugs (i.e., flupentixol and quetiapine) can also be used to treat depression.

- **Agomelatine**
- **Buspirone**
- **Lithium salts (carbonate or citrate)**
- **Mianserin**
- **Mirtazapine**
- **Trazodone**
- **Tryptophan**

The suffix '-**apine**' is not unique to the antidepressant **mirtazapine** and is one that can be applied to any tricyclic (three-ringed) chemical compound.

Antipsychotics

Antipsychotic drugs (or 'neuroleptics') are given to treat conditions such as schizophrenia and bipolar disorder. It has become common for antipsychotic drugs to be put into two broad categories: first generation (or 'typical') and second generation ('atypical'). The first (typical) antipsychotics were introduced in the 1950s (the atypical antipsychotics came later). Antipsychotics work by affecting the activity of neurotransmitters in the brain, thereby helping control psychotic feelings, hallucinations and behaviour.

First-generation antipsychotics

Developed in the 1950s, phenothiazines were the first 'first-generation' antipsychotics. They are 'antidopaminergic' – meaning that they work by inhibiting dopamine activity. The fact that dopamine transmission-blocking medicines could control schizophrenic symptoms led to the *dopamine hypothesis of schizophrenia* – the theory that schizophrenia is the result of over-stimulation of dopamine receptors in the brain (Carlsson and Lindqvist 1963, cited in Noll, 1992, p. 97). Like the phenothiazines, all first generation antipsychotics have antidopaminergic properties (see list of 'typical' antipsychotic drug groups). It is (theoretically) this dopamine-blocking quality that gives these drugs their schizophrenia-controlling power, but that same quality can also sometimes cause disorders of movement similar to those seen in Parkinson's disease (Fahn and Burke, 2010, p. 778). Flupentixol has properties that mean it can be used either as an antipsychotic or as an antidepressant. Some antipsychotic drugs can also be used to treat nausea and vomiting (see antiemetics: Chapter 7).

L**oxa**pine is a dibenz**oxa**zepine; pimozide is a diphenylbutylpiperidine; sul**piride** is a substituted benzamide; phenothiazine names end in '-**proma-zine**' or '-**perazine**' (or include the letters '**per-**' and '-**azine**'); butyrophenone names end in '-**peridol**'; while thioxanthenes end in '-**pentixol**' or '-**penthixol**':

- **Ben**peridol
- **Chlor**promazine
- **Flupentixol**
- **Fluphenazine**
- **Halo**peridol
- **Levome**promazine
- **Loxapine**
- **Per**icyazine
- **Pimozide**

- **Prochlorperazine**
- **Promazine**
- **Sulpiride**
- Trifluoperazine
- Zuclopenthixol

 Do not confuse antipsychotic drugs ending in '-**peridol**' with painkillers such as **tramadol** and **tapentadol** (see Chapter 6) or the vitamin D analogue **alfacalcidol**.

 Despite its '-**piride**' suffix, do not mistake the antidiabetes drug **glime**piride (see Chapter 8) for an antipsychotic drug of the substituted benzamide kind.

Second-generation antipsychotics

Since the 1980s, there has been a significant increase in the use of second-generation (or 'atypical') antipsychotics. When introduced it was hoped that atypical antipsychotics would be as effective as the older, typical antipsychotics but with fewer side effects. As with the typical antipsychotics, the label 'atypical' is a broad term given to a number of different drugs that share certain characteristics (see list of atypical antipsychotic drug groups). In addition to its role in treating schizophrenia, note that the second-generation antipsychotic quetiapine is also used to treat bipolar disorder and depression.

The mechanism of action of atypical antipsychotics is somewhat different from that of their typical counterparts and is not solely related to dopamine blockade. Some researchers argue that the way that atypical antipsychotics work has brought the *dopamine hypothesis of schizophrenia* (see first-generation antipsychotics) into question. Can schizophrenia really be explained solely in terms of excess dopamine activity if atypical antipsychotic drugs affect a broader range of neurotransmitters (i.e., histamine and serotonin) as well as dopamine? Others disagree and assert that dopamine (and blocking the dopamine D2 receptor in particular) remains the key factor in all antipsychotic drug activity, regardless of type. McGavock (2011, p. 105) observes that the debate about the causes of schizophrenia and about how antipsychotic drugs actually work remains unresolved. However, it is a debate that has brought useful insights into the complex and often incapacitating mental illnesses that these drugs are designed to treat.

Second-generation antipsychotics

Benzisoxazole derivative antipsychotics have names ending in '-**peridone**'; luras**idone** is a benzisothiazol derivative; amisul**pride** is a substituted benzamide; ari**piprazole** and cari**praz**ine are phenyl**piperaz**ine derivatives. The dibenzo**thia**zepines (que**tiapine**), dibenzodiazepines (cloz**apine**), dibenzo-oxepino-pyrroles (asen**apine**) and the thienobenzodiazepines (olanz**apine**) are all chemically-related, tricyclic ('three-ringed' – hence their '-**apine**' suffix) antipsychotics.

- **Amisulpride**
- **Ari**piprazole
- **Asenapine**
- **Cari**prazine
- **Clozapine**
- **Lurasidone**
- **Olanzapine**
- **Pali**peridone
- **Quetiapine**
- **Ris**peridone

Despite ending in '-**prazole**', do not mistake the atypical antipsychotic **aripiprazole** for a proton-pump inhibitor (i.e., **omeprazole**: see PPIs, Chapter 1).

Domperidone is an antiemetic (see Chapter 7), not an antipsychotic; however, its '-**peridone**' suffix is an indication that it too is a benzisoxazole derivative.

Despite its '-**pride**' suffix, do not mistake the laxative **prucalopride** (see Chapter 1) for an antipsychotic.

Benzodiazepines

Benzodiazepines are sedatives prescribed to treat insomnia, agitation or seizures (for list of those benzodiazepines used in the management of epilepsy, see section 'Antiepileptics'). The sedating effect of benzodiazepines is a result of their role in activating the inhibitory neurotransmitter GABA. Due to an association with addiction and misuse, some benzodiazepines are schedule three controlled drugs (CDs): medication that must be prescribed, administered, documented and stored according to specific legal requirements (Misuse of Drugs Act, 1971). Most benzodiazepines have names ending in '**-azepam**', '**-azam**' or '**-azolam**':

- **Alprazolam**
- **Chlordiazepoxide**
- **Clobazam**
- **Clonazepam**
- **Diazepam**
- **Flurazepam**
- **Loprazolam**
- **Lorazepam**
- **Lormetazepam**
- **Midazolam**
- **Nitrazepam**
- **Oxazepam**
- **Temazepam**

Do not mistake **nefopam** (a benzoxazocine: a non-opioid analgesic, see Chapter 6) for a benzodiazepine sedative with a name ending in '**-azepam**'.

Non-benzodiazepine sedatives

Cyclopyrrolones and imidazopyridines

Hypnotics and sedatives are medicines used to treat insomnia. There are a number of drugs that have sleep-promoting properties similar to benzodiazepines although their drug chemistry is different: the cyclo**py**rrolones and imidazo**py**ridines. Because cyclo**py**rrolones and imidazo**py**ridines both have benzodiazepine-like effects and they both act at the benzodiazepine receptor, for convenience, these drugs are often grouped together under the broad, all-encompassing label 'non-benzodiazepines'. Because most of these drugs had generic names that began with the letter **z**, they soon became colloquially referred to as the '**z-drugs**'.

Zolpidem and zopiclone are non-benzodiazepine hypnotics. Zolpidem is an imidazo**py**ridine used for the short-term management of insomnia. Zopiclone is a cyclo**pyrrolone** that has a tranquilising effect and so is prescribed as a night sedative:

- **Zolpidem**
- **Zopiclone**

Melatonin receptor agonists

Melatonin is a naturally occurring hormone that helps regulate the circadian rhythms of sleeping and waking. While not itself one of the '**z-drugs**', melatonin has similar sleep-promoting qualities:

- **Melatonin**

Antihistamines

Antihistamines (or histamine-1 receptor antagonists) are most commonly given to treat allergic disorders (Castillo et al., 2015). An allergy is a hypersensitive response to contact with an allergen (i.e., pollen, certain foods, chemicals or fabrics). It is histamine that causes the inflammatory symptoms of an allergic reaction: watery eyes, runny nose, itchy, reddened skin. Antihistamines work by stopping histamine from binding to and activating histamine-1 receptors, so bringing relief from histamine-related symptoms. They are given to treat conditions such as hay fever, conjunctivitis, sinusitis and urticaria (itchy skin).

All of the older, 'first generation' antihistamines cause drowsiness. However, this side effect can be useful and promethazine is often taken as a night sedative.

Some antihistamines (cinnarizine, cyclizine and promethazine) have antiemetic properties and so can be used to treat nausea and vomiting (see Chapter 7).

Identifying antihistamines by the letters in their names is made more complex due to variations in their name stems. However, a few recurring themes in antihistamine drug names can be noted: see following list of antihistamines (the list includes most – but not all – of the antihistamines in current use).

The designation 'antihistamine' is usually reserved for drugs that block histamine-1 receptors (H1) (see above). However, note that H2 blockers (see Chapter 1) are a particular kind of 'antihistamine' that selectively blocks the gastric acid-secreting histamine-2 (H2).

Most (but not all) antihistamines have names that end in '**-astine**', '**-rizine**', '**-izine**' or '**-tadine**':

- **Acrivastine**
- **Alimemazine**
- **Azelastine**
- **Bilastine**
- **Cetirizine**
- **Chlorphenamine**
- **Cinnarizine**
- **Clemastine**
- **Cyclizine**
- **Cyproheptadine**
- **Desloratadine**
- **Epinastine**
- **Fexofenadine**
- **Hydroxyzine**
- **Ketotifen**
- **Levocetirizine**
- **Loratadine**
- **Mizolastine**
- **Olopatadine**
- **Promethazine**
- **Rupatadine**

 Do not mistake the antiparkinsonian drug **amantadine** (see section 'Parkinson's disease drugs') for an antihistamine with a '**-tadine**'-ending name stem.

Antimuscarinics

Antimuscarinics (sometimes called 'anticholinergics') are drugs that inhibit the action of the neurotransmitter acetylcholine. Acetylcholine plays an important role in the autonomic nervous system and is involved in many processes. Acetylcholine-inhibiting drugs are used to reduce bronchial secretions, to reduce secretions of sweat or saliva or to produce an antispasmodic effect by relaxing smooth muscle (in either the gut or the bladder). Glycopyrronium and hyoscine hydrobromide are used to help dry excessive secretions in palliative care. Hyoscine hydrobromide can also be used to treat bowel colic and motion

sickness (see Chapter 7). Some antimuscarinics have bronchodilatory properties and so are used to treat respiratory disorders (see Chapter 4). Darifenacin,
fesoterodine, flavoxate, oxybutynin, propiverine, solifenacin, tolterodine and
trospium help relax an overactive bladder and so are used to treat urinary
incontinence. Propantheline can be used to treat either gastrointestinal or
genitourinary disorders. Atropine, dicycloverine and hyoscine butylbromide
exert muscle-relaxing, antispasmodic effects on gastrointestinal smooth muscle (see antispasmodics: Chapter 1). Atropine is also used to treat bradycardia, to dilate the pupils, correct refractory eye disorders and treat pesticide
poisoning. The use of atropine – first derived from the plant *Atropa belladonna*
('deadly nightshade') – has a long history: a thousand years ago the great
Islamic physician Ibn Sina catalogued its properties (along with many other
drugs) in his influential work *The Canon of Medicine*.

Note: orphenadrine, procyclidine and trihexyphenidyl are antimuscarinics
that are used in the treatment of Parkinson's disease and so are listed together
with other antiparkinsonian medicines later in this chapter.

Commonly seen antimuscarinic drug name stems include '-**clidinium**',
'-**ifenacin**', '-**terodine**', '-**tropine**' and '-**tropium**' (or variations of those
letters):

- **Aclidinium**
- **Atropine**
- **Darifenacin**
- **Dicycloverine**
- **Fesoterodine**
- **Flavoxate**
- **Glycopyrronium**
- **Homatropine**
- **Hyoscine butylbromide**
- **Hyoscine hydrobromide**
- **Ipratropium**
- **Oxybutynin**
- **Propantheline**
- **Propiverine**
- **Solifenacin**
- **Tiotropium**
- **Tolterodine**
- **Tropicamide**
- **Trospium**
- **Umeclidinium**

Do not mistake **darifenacin** and **solifenacin** for antibiotics ending in '-**cin**' (see Chapter 9) or NSAIDs with names ending in '-**fenac**' (see Chapter 6). Note: the suffix '-**verine**' is one that can be applied to any drug with smooth muscle-relaxing properties.

Parkinson's disease drugs

Parkinson's is a degenerative neurological disease. Progressive damage to a part of the brain (the substantia nigra) responsible for co-ordinating body movement results in symptoms that include tremor, bradykinesia (slowness of movement) and rigidity. Parkinson's disease causes an imbalance in the levels of two important neurotransmitters, the effect of which leaves Parkinson's disease patients with an insufficiency of dopamine (a neurotransmitter involved in movement co-ordination) and a relative excess of the complementary neurotransmitter acetylcholine.

There is no cure for Parkinson's disease, but regular medication will help control its symptoms. With antiparkinsonian drug therapy, the timing of administration is critical. If a Parkinson's disease patient is in hospital, nurses should try to give the drugs at the same time that the patient would take them at home (Sadler, 2007). If not, there is a danger that symptom control will be lost and that parkinsonian symptoms, including akinesia (an inability to initiate movement) and dyskinesia (disordered movement) will re-appear.

The aims of antiparkinsonian drug therapy are to try and replace the lacking dopamine and to counteract the relative imbalance between dopamine and acetylcholine. Parkinson's disease drug therapy is complex and often involves a variety of drug types:

Levodopa and DDI inhibitor compounds
COMT inhibitors
Dopamine receptor agonists
Monoamine oxidase-B inhibitors
Antimuscarinic antiparkinsonian drugs
Glutamate antagonists

Levodopa and DDI compounds

It is impossible to replace dopamine directly because dopamine cannot cross the blood–brain barrier. However, levodopa (the precursor to dopamine) can. Levodopa is given in combination with a DDI (dopa-decarboxylase inhibitor): either benserazide or carbidopa. The prefix '**co-**' indicates that these drugs are **co**mpounds involving two drugs **co**mbined, with the suffix '-**dopa**' reflecting the levodopa component.

Co-beneldopa (**ben**serazide/**levodopa**)
Co-careldopa (**car**bidopa/**levodopa**)

Despite its '-**dopa**' suffix, do not mistake the antihypertensive drug **methyldopa** (see Chapter 2) for an anti-Parkinson's disease drug. **Methyldopa** does have an (indirect) effect on dopamine (hence its '-**dopa**' suffix), but its effect is to inhibit dopamine activity; an effect that is the opposite of dopamine transmission-boosting anti-Parkinson's disease drugs.

COMT inhibitors

The enzyme catechol-*O*-methyltransferase (COMT) breaks down levodopa. By inhibiting this enzyme, COMT inhibitors block the conversion of levodopa to 3-*O*-methyldopa, which means that more levodopa is free to cross the blood–brain barrier for conversion into dopamine. COMT inhibitor names end in '-**capone**'.

- **Enta**capone
- **Opi**capone
- **Tol**capone

Dopamine receptor agonists

Dopamine receptor agonists are 'dopaminergic' drugs, meaning that they promote dopamine transmission. Apomorphine is given by means of subcutaneous injection. Note: bromocriptine and cabergoline can also be used to treat problems relating to lactation.

- **Apomorphine**
- **Bromocriptine**
- **Cabergoline**
- **Pergolide**
- **Pramipexole**
- **Ropinirole**
- **Rotigotine**

Despite ending in '-**morphine**', do not mistake **apomorphine** for an opioid analgesic (see Chapter 6). Although derived from morphine (hence its suffix), apomorphine has no morphine-like properties (the prefix '**apo-**' simply means 'derived from').

Monoamine oxidase-B inhibitors

Monoamine oxidase-B inhibitors selectively stop monoamine oxidase type-B (MAO-B) from breaking down dopamine, thereby making MAO-B inhibitors useful drugs in the treatment of Parkinson's disease.

- **Rasagiline**
- **Safinamide**
- **Selegiline**

Antimuscarinic antiparkinsonian drugs

In Parkinson's disease, dopamine deficiency can result in a comparative excess of the complementary neurotransmitter acetylcholine. Antimuscarinic drugs are given in Parkinson's disease to try and restore the balance between dopamine and acetylcholine levels. They can be helpful in controlling symptoms such as tremor and drooling. However, sometimes their disadvantages (dry mouth, memory problems, etc.) can outweigh their benefits, especially among the elderly.

- **Orphenadrine**
- **Procyclidine**
- **Trihexyphenidyl**

Glutamate antagonists

Amantadine was developed in the 1960s as an antiviral drug to treat influenza. However, amantadine is now rarely prescribed as a treatment for influenza (having been superseded by more effective alternatives, see antiviral agents: Chapter 9) and it is no longer recommended for that purpose. But it was later discovered that amantadine also inhibits the reuptake of dopamine, which means that it is now sometimes used as an anti-Parkinson's disease drug.

- **Amantadine**

 Do not mistake **amantadine** for an antihistamine with a name stem ending in '-**tadine**' (i.e., **desloratadine**: see section 'Antihitamines').

References

Castillo, M., Scott, N.W., Mustafa, M.Z. et al. (2015). Topical antihistamines and mast cell stabilisers for treating seasonal and perennial allergic conjunctivitis. *Cochrane Database of Systematic Reviews* [online]. Available from: doi:10.1002/14651858.CD009566. pub2.

Esiwe, C., Baillon, S., Rajkonwar, A. et al. (2016). Screening for depression in older people on acute hospital wards: the validity of the Edinburgh Depression Scale. *Age and Ageing*, 45 (4), 554–558.

Fahn, S. and Burke, R.E. (2010). Tardive dyskinesia and other neuroleptic-induced syndromes. In: Rowland, L.P. and Pedley, T.A. (eds). *Merritt's neurology*. 12th ed. Philadelphia: Lippincott Williams and Wilkins, pp. 778–781.

McGavock, H. (2011). *How drugs work: basic pharmacology for healthcare professionals*. 3rd ed. Oxford: Radcliffe Publishing Ltd.

Misuse of Drugs Act (1971). Chapter 38. London: HMSO [online]. Available from: http://www.legislation.gov.uk/ukpga/1971/38.

Noll, R. (1992). *The encyclopaedia of schizophrenia and the psychotic disorders*. New York: Facts On File.

Rossetti, A.O. (2016). Are newer AEDs better than the classic ones in the treatment of status epilepticus? *Journal of Clinical Neurophysiology*, 33 (1), 18–21.

Sadler, C. (2007). It's all in the timing. *Nursing Standard*, 21 (24), 20–21.

Drugs used in the management of pain

6

Non-opioid analgesics
Compound analgesics
Opioids analgesics
5HT-1 agonists
NSAIDs (non-steroidal anti-inflammatory drugs):
    Enolic acid class NSAIDs
    Acetic acid class NSAIDs
    Propionic acid class NSAIDs
    Fenamic acid class NSAIDs
    COX-2 inhibitor class NSAIDs

Analgesics

Analgesics (or 'painkillers') are among the most important drugs that nurses are called upon to administer. Helping to control their pain is central to your patient's quality of life. Pain-relieving drugs should be given according to an assessment of pain severity. The World Health Organisation's *Analgesic Ladder* (World Health Organisation, 1996, p. 15) advocates a structured approach to prescribing, moving up, step by step, from non-opioid analgesics (for mild pain) to increasingly stronger opioids until pain is controlled.

Non-opioid analgesics

Aspirin is now mainly prescribed for its antiplatelet properties (see Chapter 3); however, it continues to be taken as a non-prescription medicine for its original purpose: a drug for treating mild to moderate pain. Nefopam is a benzoxazocine: a centrally-acting, non-opioid analgesic given for moderate pain.

The Drug Recognition Guide, Second Edition. Mark Currivan.
© 2021 John Wiley & Sons Ltd. Published 2021 by John Wiley & Sons Ltd.

Paracetamol is a drug that has both analgesic and antipyretic (temperature-reducing) properties. In care settings paracetamol is often preferred to aspirin because it is equally effective as a painkiller while being less irritating to the gastric mucosa. Veal et al. (2014) maintains that better and regular use of paracetamol could help reduce the need for opioid prescription.

- **Aspirin**
- **Nefopam**
- **Paracetamol**

 Despite having a name ending in '-**pam**', do not mistake the painkiller **nefopam** for a benzodiazepine sedative with a name ending in '-**azepam**' (see Chapter 5).

Compound analgesics

Compound analgesics usually combine a non-opioid analgesic with a 'weaker' opioid analgesic. They are given to help control mild to moderate pain. Two different types of medication given together can produce a synergistic effect (more effective than the same drugs given separately). However, combining non-opioids and opioids in one tablet can make upward titration of the various elements within the compound more complex and can increase the possibilities for overdose. The prefix '**co-**' at the beginning of a drug name is an indication that it is a **co**mpound of two different drugs **co**mbined in the one tablet. Compound analgesics that contain **parace**t**amol** as a constituent part can be identified by the suffix '-**amol**' (note a recent name change: for reasons of clarity and safety '**co**-**dydramol**' is now to be known as '**dihydr**ocodeine with parace**tamol**'):

Co-codamol (codeine with paracetamol)
Dihydrocodeine with paracetamol

An overdose of paracetamol (i.e., more than 4 g in 24 hours) can be hepatotoxic: toxic to the liver (Heard et al., 2016). Nurses must be careful to check what drugs their patient has taken in the past 24 hours to ensure that they do not give an additional (separate) dose of paracetamol too soon after a paracetamol-containing compound analgesic has been taken.

 Note some exceptions: drugs ending in '-**amol**' that are not **paracetamol**-containing medicines: **salbutamol** (a beta-2 agonist: see Chapter 4) and **methocarbamol** (a centrally-acting muscle relaxant).

Opioid analgesics

If non-opioid analgesics – drugs used to treat mild to moderate pain – fail to bring the pain under control, it is appropriate to step up the *Analgesic Ladder* and for doctors to prescribe an opioid: a more powerful kind of analgesia derived from the opium poppy or made synthetically to have opium-like effects. The pain-relieving properties of opium have been known about since antiquity. The drug name '**codeine**' comes from the Greek word 'kodeia' (a term meaning the head of a poppy). Opioid analgesics are often described as being either 'weaker' or 'stronger'. The so-called weaker opioids (codeine phosphate and dihydrocodeine) are used to treat moderate to moderately severe pain. The weaker opioids are often included in compound analgesics (see section 'Compound analgesics') but can be given separately. If the weaker opioids fail to control the pain, it may be appropriate to step up again and for one of the stronger opioids to be prescribed.

The stronger opioids (alfentanil, fentanyl, diamorphine, morphine, oxycodone, etc.) are used to treat severe pain. Morphine, for example, is approximately 10 times stronger than codeine (Curtin, 2019, p. 561). The name '**morphine**' comes from **Morph**eus, the Greek god of dreams. The '-**codone**' part of the drug name oxy**codone** is derived from the word '**cod**eine'. Opioid analgesics tend to cause constipation and can depress the respiratory rate. The stronger opioids are controlled drugs (CDs): medication subject to specific legal requirements about how they are prescribed, administered, documented and stored. See following list of most (but not all) opioid analgesics, both weaker and stronger.

The prefix '**a-**' is Ancient Greek for 'without' (i.e., as in the word '**a**septic'); '**dol**or' is the Latin word for pain: so the suffix '-**adol**' simply means 'without pain'. '**Papaver**' is Latin for 'poppy', hence the name **papaver**etum.

- **Alfentanil**
- **Bupren**orphine
- **Codeine phosphate**
- **Dia**morphine
- **Dihydrocodeine**
- **Dipipanone**
- **Fentanyl**
- **Hydro**morph**one**
- **Methad**one
- **Morphine** sulfate
- **Oxycodone**
- **Papaver**etum

- **Pentazocine**
- **Pethidine**
- **Remifentanil**
- **Sufentanil**
- **Tapentadol**
- **Tramadol**

Note drugs ending in '-**dol**' (but not '-**adol**') that are not painkillers: **benperidol**, **droperidol** and **haloperidol** (see antipsychotics in Chapter 5 and antiemetics in Chapter 7) and the vitamin D analogue **alfacalcidol**.

5HT-1 agonists

5HT-1 agonists are drugs given to treat migraine. Serotonin is a neurotransmitter that plays a role in many of the body's physical and emotional processes. Medication that enhances serotonin transmission to particular receptors are known as serotonin agonists, whereas medicines that inhibit serotonin transmission are called serotonin antagonists. The serotonin antagonists include drugs used to treat nausea and vomiting (see Chapter 7); while serotonin transmission-enhancing drugs can include those used to treat constipation (see Chapter 1), depression (see Chapter 5) and – in this instance – migraine. The full chemical name for serotonin is 5-hydroxy**trypta**mine (often abbreviated to 5HT). When the neurotransmitter serotonin-1 (5HT-1) binds to serotonin-1 receptors, it constricts the cranial blood vessels, thereby reducing the inflammation that causes the symptoms of a migraine attack (headache, photophobia, etc.). 5HT-1 agonists were first introduced in the 1990s and their effectiveness meant that migraine sufferers often preferred them to previously used medicines for migraine (Robbins, 2002). The '**triptans**' (as they soon began to be called) were the first anti-migraine drugs that tried to treat the underlying cause of migraine rather than merely trying to alleviate its symptoms.

- **Almotriptan**
- **Eletriptan**
- **Frovatriptan**
- **Naratriptan**
- **Rizatriptan**
- **Sumatriptan**
- **Zolmitriptan**

Non-steroidal anti-inflammatory drugs (NSAIDs)

Non-steroidal anti-inflammatory drugs (NSAIDs) are, as their name indicates, anti-inflammatory agents other than those of the steroid kind. NSAIDs work by blocking the enzyme cyclo-oxygenase (COX). Blocking COX inhibits prostaglandin synthesis. Prostaglandins are hormone-like substances involved in transmitting pain signals to the nervous system. The reduction in pain impulse transmission that results from COX inhibition can make NSAIDs highly effective analgesics. However, reducing prostaglandin levels can have unwanted side effects. In particular, because prostaglandins also help protect the mucosal lining of the stomach, NSAIDs can increase the risk of gastric ulceration. For this reason, NSAIDs should be used cautiously in people known or considered to be at risk of gastrointestinal bleeding (Davies, 2018, p. 34).

NSAIDs can be subdivided into the enolic acid, acetic acid, propionic acid, fenamic acid and COX-2 inhibitor classes. Most NSAIDs are 'non-selective' and work by inhibiting both COX-1 and COX-2 enzymes; whereas COX-2 inhibitors are 'selective' and primarily affect COX-2 enzymes (inhibiting different COX enzymes has different effects). Note: aspirin can also be classified as an NSAID (see aspirin sections in Chapters 3 and 6).

Enolic acid class NSAIDs

NSAIDs of the enolic acid class can be recognised by names that end in '-**oxicam**':

- **Meloxicam**
- **Piroxicam**
- **Tenoxicam**

Acetic acid, propionic acid and fenamic acid class NSAIDs

The **ac**etic acid and **pro**pionic acid class NSAIDs have names that end in or include the letters '-**ac**', '-**fenac**', '-(**bu**)**profen**' and '-**metacin**':

- **Aceclofenac**
- **Dexibuprofen**
- **Dexketoprofen**
- **Diclofenac**
- **Etodolac**
- **Felbinac**
- **Flurbiprofen**
- **Ibuprofen**

- **Indometacin**
- **Ketoprofen**
- **Ketorolac**
- **Mefenamic acid**
- **Nabumetone**
- **Naproxen**
- **Nepafenac**
- **Sulindac**
- **Tiaprofenic acid**

Do not mistake the NSAID **indometacin** for an antibiotic ending in '-**mycin**' (see Chapter 9) or an antimuscarinic ending in '-**ifenacin**' (see Chapter 5). Also, do not mistake the antihistamine **ketotifen** (see Chapter 5) for an NSAID ending in '-**profen**'.

Cyclo-oxygenase (COX)-2 inhibitors

COX-2 inhibitors are a class of NSAID analgesic with a mode of action that is more selective than the other NSAID classes. Selective COX-2 inhibitors were designed to have an effect on the enzyme COX-2 and tried to avoid affecting COX-1 (COX-1 enzyme inhibition being primarily responsible for the effect that NSAIDs have on the gastro-protective prostaglandins). By targeting COX-2, it was hoped that COX-2 inhibitors would be less likely to have the negative gastrointestinal side effects (the increased risk of gastric ulcer) associated with the other, non-selective NSAIDs.

As the twenty-first century began, COX-2 inhibitors were being hailed in the media as a breakthrough in pain management. Selective COX-2 inhibitors were, for a brief period, thought to possess all of the pain-relieving benefits of the other, non-selective NSAIDs without any of their troublesome, ulcer-causing side effects. However, in 2004, the COX-2 inhibitor rofecoxib was withdrawn due to concerns about a completely different safety issue: an increased risk of myocardial infarction and stroke (Angell, 2005, p. 265). COX-2 inhibitors are now given in preference to non-selective NSAIDs only when the risk of a cardiovascular disease event is deemed to be low.

NSAIDs of the COX-2 inhibitor class have names that end in the letters '-**coxib**':

- **Celecoxib**
- **Etoricoxib**
- **Parecoxib**

References

Angell, M. (2005). *The truth about drug companies: how they deceive us and what to do about it*. New York: Random House Paperback Edition.

Curtin, J. (2019). Pain management. In: Tadman, M., Roberts, D. and Foulkes, M. (eds). *Oxford handbook of cancer nursing*. 2nd ed. Oxford: Oxford University Press, pp. 549–568.

Davies, E. (2018). Safe and effective management of analgesics in patients presenting to hospital with acute illness. *Nursing Standard*, 33 (9), 31–37.

Heard, K., Green, J.L., Anderson, V. et al. (2016). Paracetamol (acetaminophen) protein adduct concentrations during therapeutic dosing. *British Journal of Clinical Pharmacology*, 81 (3), 562–568.

Robbins, L. (2002). Triptans versus analgesics. *Headache The Journal of Head and Face Pain*, 42 (9), 903–907 [online]. Wiley Online Library. Available from: doi: 10.1046/j.1526-4610.2002.02211.x.

Veal, F.C., Bereznicki, L.R., Thompson, A.J. et al. (2014). Pharmacological management of pain in Australian aged care facilities. *Age and Ageing*, 43 (6), 851–856.

World Health Organisation (1996). *Cancer pain relief: with a guide to opioid availability*. 2nd ed. Geneva: World Health Organisation.

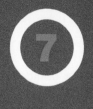

Antiemetics: drugs used in the management of nausea and vomiting

Analogues of histamine
Antihistamine antiemetics
Antimuscarinic antiemetics
Dopamine receptor antagonists
5HT-3 receptor antagonists
Neurokinin-1 receptor antagonists
Phenothiazines

Note: antimuscarinics are drugs that can also be used to treat gastrointestinal disorders (see Chapter 1), respiratory disorders (see Chapter 4), bradycardia, genitourinary disorders and Parkinson's disease (see Chapter 5).

Note: phenothiazines are also used in the treatment of mental illness (see Chapter 5).

Antiemetics

Nausea is a distressing and debilitating symptom that can have a serious impact on quality of life, particularly in those nearing the end of their life (Webb, 2017).

The Drug Recognition Guide, Second Edition. Mark Currivan.
© 2021 John Wiley & Sons Ltd. Published 2021 by John Wiley & Sons Ltd.

Analogues of histamine

The histamine analogue betahistine is used to treat vestibular disorders such as Ménière's disease and vertigo. Betahistine improves the vestibular blood flow, thereby reducing nauseating pressure in the inner ear. Do not mistake betahistine for an antihistamine. Antihistamines (see below and see antihistamine section in Chapter 5) block the secretion and action of histamine, whereas betahistine is designed to have a **histamine**-like effect on the inner ear.

- **Betahistine**

Antihistamine antiemetics

Some antihistamines have properties that make them particularly effective as antiemetics. Note that there are two different kinds of promethazine: promethazine hydrochloride and promethazine teoclate; both can be used to treat nausea and vomiting, with the latter being the longer-acting of the two:

- **Cinnarizine**
- **Cyclizine**
- **Promethazine**

Do not confuse the antihistamine **promethazine** with the antipsychotic drug **promazine** (see Chapter 5).

Antimuscarinic antiemetics

The antimuscarinic drug hyoscine hydrobromide is used to treat motion sickness (also see antimuscarinic drugs section in Chapter 5).

- **Hyoscine hydrobromide**

Dopamine receptor antagonists

The dopamine-blocking properties of antipsychotics (see antipsychotic drugs section in Chapter 5) can make them – or their derivatives – equally effective in treating nausea and vomiting. Dopamine receptor antagonists are both the oldest and most commonly given antiemetics (Smith et al., 2012). Domperidone, droperidol, haloperidol and metoclopramide are (like phenothiazine antiemetics) all anti-sickness drugs derived from – or chemically related to – antipsychotic agents (haloperidol can be used to treat either condition). Dom**peridone** is an antiemetic, not an antipsychotic, but it has enough in common with the benzisoxazole antipsychotics (i.e., ris**peridone**) to share the same '-**peridone**' name stem. Droperidol and haloperidol are butyrophenones; while metoclopramide is a benzamide derivative (and therefore structurally related to the substituted benzamide group of antipsychotic drugs).

- **Dom**peridone
- **Dro**peridol
- **Halo**peridol
- **Metoclopramide**

5HT-3 receptor antagonists

5HT (5-hydroxytryptamine) (better known as serotonin) is a neurotransmitter. When serotonin binds to specific 5HT receptors around the body, it triggers particular responses. 5HT-3 receptors are involved in stimulating the vomiting reflex (Johnston et al., 2014). 5HT-3 antagonists are drugs that stop serotonin from binding to 5HT-3 receptors, thereby helping to suppress feelings of nausea. Their name stem (derived from the word **seroton**in) reflects their mode of action:

- **Granisetron**
- **Ondansetron**
- **Palonosetron**

Do not mistake **dantron** (a simulant laxative) for a 5HT-3 antagonist ending in '-**setron**'. **Dantron** is used as a component part of the compound laxatives **co-danthramer** and **co-danthrusate** (see Chapter 1).

Neurokinin-1 receptor antagonists

Neurokinin are message-transmitting neuropeptides. Neurokinin-1 receptor antagonists are drugs used to help alleviate the severe nausea associated with chemotherapy (Viale, 2005). They are usually given together with a 5HT-3 antagonist.

- **Aprepitant**
- **Fosaprepitant**
- **Netupitant (given with palonosetron)**
- **Rolapitant**

Phenothiazines

The phenothiazines are a class of medicines initially developed to treat schizophrenia (see Chapter 5). Some phenothiazines – in addition to their antipsychotic properties – can also be used as anti-sickness agents (Hardy et al., 2015, p. 666). Phenothiazines are dopamine antagonists (see other dopamine receptor-inhibiting antiemetics earlier in this chapter) and their effectiveness as antiemetics is due to their action in blocking nausea-inducing dopamine stimulation in the chemoreceptor trigger zone part of the brain. However, inhibiting dopamine transmission can occasionally cause extrapyramidal side effects, including pseudo-parkinsonian disorders of movement and muscle co-ordination (although these – usually rare – side effects tend to resolve once the medication is discontinued).

Finn et al. (2005) observes that buccal administration (placing a dissolvable tablet between the upper lip and gum and leaving it to dissolve) of an antiemetic drug can enhance its effectiveness. Phenothiazine drug names end in '-**promazine**' or '-**perazine**':

- Chlor**promazine**
- Levome**promazine**
- Pro**chlorperazine**
- Trifluo**perazine**

Note: the antihistamine **promethazine** is chemically related to the phenothiazines (hence the similarity in the letters in its name) but – anti-sickness apart – it does not share the same properties.

References

Finn, A., Collins, J., Voyksner, R. et al. (2005). Bioavailability and metabolism of prochlorperazine administered via the buccal and oral delivery route. *Journal of Clinical Pharmacology*, 45 (12), 1383–1390 [online]. Wiley Online Library. Available from: doi: 10.1177/0091270005281044.

Hardy, J.R., Glare, P., Yates, P. et al. (2015). Palliation of nausea and vomiting. In: Cherny, N.I., Fallon, M.T., Kaasa, S. et al. (eds). *Oxford textbook of palliative medicine*. 5th ed. Oxford: Oxford University Press, pp. 661–674.

Johnston, K.D., Lu, Z. and Rudd, J.A. (2014). Looking beyond 5-HT(3) receptors: a review of the wider role of serotonin in the pharmacology of nausea and vomiting. *European Journal of Pharmacology*, 722, 13–25 [online]. Available from: doi: 10.1016/j.ejphar.2013.10.014.

Smith, H.S., Cox, L.R. and Smith, B.R. (2012). Dopamine receptor antagonists. *Annals of Palliative Medicine*, 1 (2) [online]. Available from: http://www.apm.amegroups.com/article/view/1039/1266.

Viale, P.H. (2005). Integrating aprepitant and palonosetron into clinical practice: a role for the new antiemetics. *Clinical Journal of Oncology Nursing*, 9 (1), 77–84.

Webb, A. (2017). Management of nausea and vomiting in patients with advanced cancer at the end of life. *Nursing Standard*, 32 (10), 53–63.

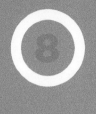

Diabetes drug therapy and other medicines that affect the endocrine system

Drugs that affect hormone, hormone-like and enzymatic activity
Insulins
Antidiabetic drugs
Bisphosphonates
Corticosteroids
Phosphodiesterase inhibitors
Prostaglandin analogues

 Note: sex hormones and hormone antagonists are another drug category that work by affecting hormonal activity. However, because of their particular role, they are listed in Chapter 10.

Insulins

Diabetes is a disorder in which the person has difficulty in maintaining their blood glucose levels within normal range (4–7 mmol/L). The two main types of diabetes are type 1 (insulin deficient) and type 2 (insulin resistant: see Section 'Antidiabetic drugs'). Insulin is a hormone secreted by the pancreas that lowers blood glucose levels. For people with type 1 diabetes regular treatment with insulin is essential. It is all too easy to take insulin for granted and to forget the impact that medicinal insulin made when it was introduced.

The Drug Recognition Guide, Second Edition. Mark Currivan.
© 2021 John Wiley & Sons Ltd. Published 2021 by John Wiley & Sons Ltd.

The story of the first insulin injections is one of the most often repeated tales in medicine, but it is worth re-telling if only to highlight the power and importance of this drug. Before the development of medicinal insulin in the 1920s, there was no effective treatment for type 1 diabetes and most people with the condition died in childhood. Diabetes wards a century ago were hospice-like places full of terminally ill children, often with parents in attendance, waiting for the inevitable to happen. A team at Toronto General Hospital in Canada began extracting insulin from animals with the intention of utilising it as a drug. One day in January 1922 Dr Frederick Banting and medical student Charles Best began injecting children (some of whom were lapsing into a diabetic coma and were close to death) with their new insulin extract. They made their way along the ward, going from bed to bed, from child to child. The effect of insulin was as rapid as it was dramatic. By the time Banting and Best had reached the other end of the ward, the first children that had been given insulin were already coming out of coma. The excitement and joy that must have swept through the ward that day must have been unforgettable to all who witnessed it.

The drug used to treat type 1 diabetes is insulin. Insulins can be put into four broad groups:

Short-acting insulins
Intermediate-acting insulins
Long-acting insulins
Biphasic insulins

Short-acting insulins

Short-acting insulins act quickly but their blood glucose-lowering effect lasts for only a relatively short period of time (up to 8 hours). Short-acting insulins can be given subcutaneously or intravenously depending on patient need.

- **Insulin aspart**
- **Insulin glulisine**
- **Insulin lispro**
- **Soluble (neutral) insulin**

Intermediate and long-acting insulins

Intermediate and long-acting insulins have a slower onset but longer duration of action (up to 24 hours or even longer). They can only be given subcutaneously.

- **Insulin degludec**
- **Insulin detemir**

- **Insulin glargine**
- **Insulin zinc suspension**
- **Isophane insulin**
- **Protamine zinc insulin**

Biphasic insulins

Biphasic insulins are compounds that contain a mixture of both short and intermediate-acting insulin. Like intermediate and long-acting insulin, biphasic insulin can only be given subcutaneously (not intravenously).

- **Biphasic aspart/aspart protamine**
- **Biphasic lispro/lispro protamine**
- **Biphasic soluble insulin/isophane**

Biphasic insulin is often given by means of metered insulin 'pens'. The biphasic (two-phased) nature of these insulin compounds can be seen in brand names that utilise parts of the word '**comb**ination' or '**mix**ture'. Insulin pens that contain a mixture of short and intermediate-acting insulin include: **Humulin® M3** (**M** for **m**ixture and **3** for 3/10th short-acting and, therefore, 7/10th intermediate-acting ins**ulin**); **Insuman® Comb 15** (15% short-acting and 85% intermediate-acting **insul**in) and **NovoMix® 30** (30% short-acting and 70% intermediate-acting insulin). All insulin (whether short, intermediate, long-acting or biphasic) is either **hum**an insulin, a hu**man** insulin analogue, or animal insulin (porcine or bovine). Insulin can only be given by injection: it cannot be given in tablet form. This is because insulin is essentially protein and its glucose-lowering action would be neutralised by protein-consuming enzymes in the stomach. Insulin is usually prescribed using the insulin's brand name and always prescribed in 'units'. Always check the concentration of insulin before giving. The concentration of insulin most commonly seen is 100 units in 1 mL. However, be aware that there are much stronger concentrations of 300 units in 1 mL (and even 500 units in 1 mL).

Antidiabetic drugs

For some people with type 2 diabetes, lifestyle changes (adhering to a diabetic diet, increased exercise, etc.) may be enough to control their illness; for others, antidiabetic drugs (blood glucose-lowering medication) will be required.

Due to factors such as an ageing population, obesity and a 'Westernised' lifestyle, the prevalence of type 2 diabetes around the world is increasing. The number of adults with diabetes in the world is predicted to rise from approximately 450 million people in 2017 to almost 700 million by 2045 (Cho et al.,

2018). It is estimated that half of all the adults in the world with diabetes are undiagnosed and so are likely to be both unaware of their illness and untreated. Because of the health implications for individuals and the cost implications for healthcare systems worldwide, the term 'diabetes epidemic' is frequently used. In the USA, for example, it has been predicted that the overall cost of diabetes care will more than double in the next 20 years. However, this increase in the prevalence of diabetes is being mirrored by an increase in the research effort to develop a growing number of new drugs and new ways to treat diabetes (Shomali, 2012).

The antidiabetic drugs used to treat type 2 diabetes can be put into a few broad categories: drugs that increase the secretion of insulin (the 'secreta-gogues': DPP-4 inhibitors, GLP-1 agonists, meglitinides and sulfonylureas); drugs that increase sensitivity to insulin (the 'sensitizers': biguanides and TZDs); drugs that reduce the absorption of carbohydrates in the gastrointestinal system (alpha-glucosidase inhibitors) and glycosuria-promoting drugs that make the kidneys excrete glucose in the urine (SGLT2 inhibitors).

Alpha-glucosidase inhibitors

Alpha-glucosidase is a digestive enzyme involved in the breakdown and utilisation of carbohydrate. By blocking this enzyme, acarbose slows down the digestion of starches and other **carb**ohydrates and so reduces the rate of glucose absorption.

- **Acarbose**

Biguanides

The wildflower *Galega officinalis* (goat's rue or French lilac) has been used as a herbal remedy for diabetes for hundreds of years. In the 1950s, **guanid**ine – the active ingredient in *G. officinalis* – was utilised to develop the modern antidiabetic agents known as bi**guanid**es. Biguanides reduce blood glucose levels by reducing glucose production in the liver and by increasing sensitivity to insulin. They do not increase insulin secretion and so are less likely to cause the kind of hypoglycaemia or weight gain that can sometimes occur with the insulin-depleting sulfonylurea antidiabetic drugs. Metformin has a proven track record in helping people with type 2 diabetes maintain control over their illness, and it has become a cornerstone of antidiabetic drug therapy. It should, however, be used with caution in people with chronic kidney disease (CKD). Biguanides have names ending with the suffix '-**formin**':

- **Metformin**

Dipeptidylpeptidase-4 inhibitors

The incretin GLP-1 (**gl**ucagon-**l**ike **p**eptide-1) is an intestinal hormone that stimulates insulin secretion. GLP-1 incretins are metabolised soon after their release and rendered inactive by an enzyme called DPP-4 (dipeptidylpeptidase-4). DPP-4 inhibitors block the action of the DPP-4 enzyme, prolonging the action of GLP-1 incretins and so increasing insulin secretion.

- **Alogliptin**
- **Linagliptin**
- **Saxagliptin**
- **Sitagliptin**
- **Vildagliptin**

Glucagon-like peptide-1 agonists

Glucagon-like pep**tide**-1 receptor agonists are incretin 'mimetics': drugs that mimic the action and effects of GLP-1 incretins (see DPP-4 inhibitors). They are given by means of subcutaneous injection. Incretin-based therapy is effective and its use is increasing (Nauck, 2013).

- **Dulaglutide**
- **Exenatide**
- **Liraglutide**
- **Lixisenatide**
- **Semaglutide**

Note: teduglutide is a GLP-2 analogue used in the treatment of short bowel syndrome. Do not mistake it for an antidiabetic agent of the GLP-1 agonist kind.

Meglitinides

Meglitinides should be taken just before a meal – if a meal is delayed – the dose can be delayed. They are designed to trigger an increase in insulin secretion at times when it coincides with times of heightened blood glucose levels (i.e., mealtimes). They are fast but short-acting (Owens, 2004). Because of the targeting in the timing of insulin secretion, they are thought less likely to cause the kind of hypoglycaemia that can sometimes occur with the sulfonylurea antidiabetic agents. You can recognise meglitinides by names ending in '**-glinide**':

- **Nateglinide**
- **Repaglinide**

Sodium-glucose (linked) co-transporter 2 inhibitors

Sodium-glucose linked co-transporter 2 (SGLT2) are proteins involved in the reabsorption of glucose in the kidneys. Sodium-glucose co-transporter 2 inhibitors are 'glyco**sur**ics', a type of antidiabetic drug that works by inhibiting SGLT2, thereby promoting glyco**suria**: the intentional excretion of glucose in the **uri**ne (Mudaliar et al., 2015). Sodium glucose co-transporter 2 inhibitor drug names end in '**-gliflozin**':

- **Canagliflozin**
- **Dapagliflozin**
- **Empagliflozin**
- **Ertugliflozin**

Sulfonylureas

Sulfonylureas work by stimulating the pancreas to secrete more insulin. While metformin (see Section 'Biguanides') is the drug of choice for people with type 2 diabetes who are overweight, a sulfonylurea is often preferred for those who are not. Most sulfonylureas have names that begin with the prefix '**gli-**':

- **Glibenclamide**
- **Gliclazide**
- **Glimepiride**
- **Glipizide**
- **Tolbutamide**

Thiazolidinediones

Thiazolidined**iones** (TZDs) work by affecting receptors involved in the metabolism of fatty acids and glucose, resulting in a decrease in insulin resistance and a corresponding increase in sensitivity to insulin. Although sometimes given on its own, pioglitazone is more often used in combination with other antidiabetic agents. TZDs have names ending in '**-glitazone**':

- **Pioglitazone**

Note: a feature common to many hypoglycaemic (blood glucose-lowering) medicines: names containing the letters '**gli**': DPP-4 inhibitors (i.e., **saxagliptin**), meglitinides (i.e., **repaglinide**), SGLT2 inhibitors (i.e., **canagliflozin**), sulfonylureas (i.e., **gliclazide**) and thiazolidinediones (**pioglitazone**).

Bisphosphonates

Bone is subject to a gradual but continual process of resorption and renewal: osteoclasts break down old bone material, which results in calcium being released into the bloodstream; osteoblasts, meanwhile, are constantly making new bone (Rang et al., 2016, pp. 444–445). The bone resorption and bone-making process can be affected by numerous factors (the menopause, vitamin-D deficiency, steroid therapy, etc.) and bone density can be lost. Consequently, bones become more brittle and prone to fracture.

Bisphosphonates are drugs given to prevent or treat osteoporosis. They work by inhibiting the action of the osteoclasts involved in bone resorption. This slows down the rate of bone turnover, giving the bone-forming osteoblasts more time and so preserves bone density. Some bisphosphonates are prescribed to treat hypercalcaemia (high levels of calcium in the blood). As old bone tissue is broken down by osteoclasts, calcium is released into the circulation. The osteoclast-inhibiting action of bisphosphonates means that, as well as preserving bone density, they can also exert a calcium-lowering effect that can be utilised to treat hypercalcaemia. Bisphosphonates have names ending in either '-**dronate**' or '-**dronic acid**':

- **Alendronic acid**
- **Ibandronic acid**
- **Pamidronate disodium**
- **Risedronate sodium**
- **Sodium clodronate**
- **Zoledronic acid**

Corticosteroids

Natural corticosteroids are hormones released by the adrenal cortex. They are involved in many biological processes, including the inflammatory and immune responses and in the regulation of metabolism and electrolyte balance.

Synthetic corticosteroids ('steroids') are drugs given to treat inflammation (i.e., in Crohn's disease or ulcerative colitis); some are used to treat autoimmune or allergic disorders; others are given as hormone replacement therapy. The corticosteroids dexamethasone and prednisolone are sometimes used in cancer therapy. Corticosteroids suppress the body's immune system. Sometimes immunosuppression is the intended purpose (i.e., when given to treat autoimmune disorders or to prevent the rejection of a transplanted organ), at other times it may simply be an unintended consequence of steroid therapy. Dexamethasone has proved effective in suppressing hypersensitive immune reactions to the virus COVID-19. Steroids are well-known for their potential to cause side effects, including osteoporosis, weight gain and elevated blood glucose levels. Corticosteroids can be given in a variety of ways: by mouth, intravenously, topically or by inhalation. The inhaled corticosteroids (beclometasone, budesonide, ciclesonide, fluticasone and mometasone) are used in the treatment of asthma and COPD and work by reducing inflammation in the respiratory tract (see Chapter 4). Some respiratory conditions may require treatment with steroid tablets (i.e., prednisolone). Topical steroids, applied directly to the skin in the form of ointments or creams, are used in the management of dermatological conditions such as eczema (Lawton, 2009). The list that follows includes most – but not all – of the corticosteroids in current use.

Corticosteroid drug names include the letters '-**cort**', '-**metasone**', '-**sone**', '-(**s**)**olone**' and '-**sonide**':

- Alclometasone
- Beclometasone
- Betamethasone
- Budesonide
- Ciclesonide
- Clobetasol
- Clobetasone
- Deflazacort
- Dexamethasone
- Diflucortolone
- Fludrocortisone
- Fludroxycortide
- Flumetasone
- Fluocinolone
- Fluocortolone

- **Fluticasone**
- **Hydrocortisone**
- **Methylprednisolone**
- **Mometasone**
- **Prednisolone**
- **Triamcinolone**

 Note: the name stem '**-olone**' can also be seen in some sex hormone names (i.e., the oestrogen **tibolone**).

Phosphodiesterase inhibitors

Phosphodiesterase inhibitors are drugs that block the action of phosphodiesterase enzymes. There are 11 known types of phosphodiesterase, with different phosphodiesterase enzymes involved in helping regulate different physiological processes. As a result, drugs that inhibit specific phosphodiesterase (PDE) enzymes can be used to treat a remarkably diverse array of medical conditions.

The PDE inhibitor dipyridamole (see Chapter 3) works as an antiplatelet agent and is given to prevent thrombosis or stroke. Anagrelide is a PDE type-3 inhibitor (see Chapter 3) used in the treatment of thrombocythaemia. Cilostazol dilates the blood vessels and is used to treat claudication. PDE also plays a role in helping regulate heart muscle contractions, hence the use of the PDE type-3 inhibitors enoximone and milrinone in heart failure to increase the force of the heart's contractions.

The PDE type-4 inhibitor roflumilast has anti-inflammatory properties that are useful in treating respiratory disorders (see Chapter 4). Apremilast is a PDE type-4 inhibitor given to treat psoriatic arthritis.

Papaverine is a PDE type-10 inhibitor used as an ingredient in combination with other medicines. The suffix '**-verine**' indicates a medicine that has smooth muscle-relaxing properties (see antispasmodics: Chapter 1). The Latin word for poppy (the traditional source for opium) is '**papaver**'. While **papaverine** is not itself an opioid analgesic, it is derived from an opium alkaloid and is – together with morphine and codeine – a component part of the analgesic **papaveretum** (see opioid analgesics: Chapter 6).

When research began into the medicinal properties of drugs that selectively block the action of PDE type-5 enzymes, it was thought that they might prove useful in treating angina – but they did not. Unexpectedly they were found to be effective treatments for erectile dysfunction and pulmonary arterial hypertension. PDE type-5 inhibitors cause a targeted dilation of the blood vessels supplying the penis with blood. The first PDE type-5 inhibitor was sildenafil (perhaps better known by its brand name Viagra®), and it soon became one of the most widely reported and media-debated new drugs of the 1990s. The blood vessel-dilating properties of PDE type-5 inhibitors also make them useful in treating pulmonary arterial hypertension. Selective PDE type-5 inhibitors have generic names ending in '-**afil**':

- **Anagrelide**
- **Apremilast**
- **Avanafil**
- **Cilostazol**
- **Dipyridamole**
- **Enoximone**
- **Milrinone**
- **Papaverine**
- **Roflumilast**
- **Sildenafil**
- **Tadalafil**
- **Vardenafil**

Note: apremilast is not an anti-**ast**hmatic agent (despite its '-**ast**' suffix); it does, however, have anti-inflammatory properties.

Prostaglandin analogues

Prostaglandin analogues are drugs that are made to act like natural prostaglandins and which have similarly diverse properties. Bimatoprost, latanoprost, tafluprost and travoprost are used to treat glaucoma. Iloprost has antihypertensive properties and is given to treat pulmonary arterial hypertension. Alprostadil is a vaso**dila**tor given to treat erectile dysfunction. Epoprostenol (see Chapter 3) has anticoagulant properties and is given to prevent clotting in extracorporeal lines during haemodialysis sessions. Carboprost, dinoprostone, gemeprost and misoprostol are used in obstetric medicine (in the induction of labour, postpartum haemorrhage and in termination of pregnancy). Because NSAIDs (see Chapter 6) can affect prostaglandin levels, the prostaglandin analogue misoprostol (which has a gastro-protective effect) is sometimes given in addition to an NSAID to prevent NSAID-induced gastric ulceration. Prostaglandin analogues feature the letters '-**prost**-' in their names:

- **Alprostadil**
- **Bimatoprost**
- **Carboprost**
- **Dinoprostone**
- **Epoprostenol**
- **Gemeprost**
- **Iloprost**
- **Latanoprost**
- **Misoprostol**
- **Tafluprost**
- **Travoprost**

References

Cho, N.H., Shaw, J.E., Karuranga, S. et al. (2018). I.D.F. (International Diabetes Federation) Diabetes Atlas: global estimates of diabetes prevalence for 2017 and projections for 2045. *Diabetes Research and Clinical Practice*, 138, 271–281 [online]. Available from: doi: 10.1016/j.diabres.2018.02.023.

Lawton, S. (2009). Assessing and treating adult patients with eczema. *Nursing Standard*, 23 (43), 49–56.

Mudaliar, S., Polidori, D., Zambrowicz, B. et al. (2015). Sodium–glucose cotransporter inhibitors: effects on renal and intestinal glucose transport: from bench to bedside. *Diabetes Care*, 38 (12), 2344–2354.

Nauck, M.A. (2013). A critical analysis of the clinical use of incretin-based therapies: the benefits by far outweigh the potential risks. *Diabetes Care*, 36 (7), 2126–2132.

Owens, D.R. (2004). Repaglinide – prandial glucose regulator: a new class of oral antidiabetic drugs. *Diabetic Medicine*, 15, (Supplement 4), S28–S36 [online]. Wiley Online Library. Available from: doi: 10.1002/(sici)1096-9136(1998120)15:4+<S28::aid-dia748>3.3.

Rang, H.P., Ritter, J.M., Flower, R.J. et al. (2016). *Rang and Dale's pharmacology*. 8th ed. Churchill Livingstone: Elsevier

Shomali, M. (2012). Diabetes treatment in 2025: can scientific advances keep pace with prevalence? *Therapeutic Advances in Endocrinology and Metabolism*, 3 (5), 163–173 [online] Available from: doi: 10.1177/2042018812465639.

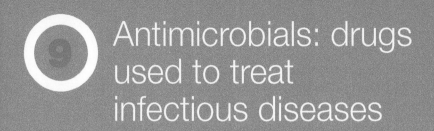

Antimicrobials: drugs used to treat infectious diseases

Antibacterials ('antibiotics')

Aminoglycosides
Cephalosporins
Folic acid inhibitors
Lipopeptides and glycopeptides
Macrocyclic antibiotics
Nitrofuran derivatives
Oxazolidinones
Quinolones
Sulfonamides
Tetracyclines and glycylcyclines

Carbapenems
Compound antibiotics
Lincosamides

Macrolides
Nitroimidazoles
Penicillins
Rifamycins

Antifungals

Echinocandin class
Imidazole class
Polyene class
Triazole class

Antivirals

Fusion (entry) inhibitors
HCV inhibitors
Interferons
Integrase inhibitors
Neuraminidase inhibitors
Nucleoside analogues
Nucleotide analogues
Nucleoside reverse transcriptase inhibitors

The Drug Recognition Guide, Second Edition. Mark Currivan.
© 2021 John Wiley & Sons Ltd. Published 2021 by John Wiley & Sons Ltd.

Non-nucleoside reverse transcriptase inhibitors
Phosphonic acid derivatives
Protease inhibitors (hepatitis C and HIV-affecting)

Antibacterials

Antibacterials (commonly called 'antibiotics') are drugs given to treat a bacterial infection (as distinct from a fungal or viral infection). The emergence of effective antibacterial agents, in particular, Fleming's discovery of penicillin and its subsequent development by Florey, Chain, Heatley and others, proved to be the most important pharmaceutical breakthrough of the twentieth century. More lives have been saved because of treatment with antibiotics than with any other type of medicine in history. There are many types of antibacterial agent, with specific types required to treat specific kinds of bacteria. Listed in this section are most (but not all) of the antibacterials in current use.

Aminoglycosides

Aminoglycosides have a broad spectrum of activity and are used to treat both Gram-negative and Gram-positive organisms. Aminoglycosides have names ending with '-**kacin**', '-**micin**' or '-**mycin**'. The suffix '-**cin**' is one that is common to many antibacterials.

- **Amikacin**
- **Gentamicin**
- **Neomycin**
- **Streptomycin**
- **Tobramycin**

Note a few exceptions – drugs ending in '-**cin**' that are not antibacterial agents: the antimuscarinic drugs **darifenacin** and **solifenacin** (see Chapter 5); the NSAID **indometacin** (see Chapter 6); the topical analgesic **capsaicin** and the obstetric medicines **carbetocin** and **oxytocin**.

Carbapenems

Carbapenems are beta-lactam antibacterial agents. Because an enzyme in the kidney inactivates imipenem, it is given in combination with cilastatin (an enzyme inhibitor). Carbapenems end in '-**penem**':

- **Ertapenem**
- **Imipenem with cilastatin**
- **Meropenem**

 Despite ending in '-**statin**', do not mistake **cilastatin** for a cholesterol-lowering drug (see statins: Chapter 3).

Cephalosporins

Cephalosporins are used to treat septicaemia, meningitis, peritonitis, pneumonia and infections of the biliary and urinary tracts.

- **Cefaclor**
- **Cefadroxil**
- **Cefalexin**
- **Cefixime**
- **Cefotaxime**
- **Cefradine**
- **Ceftaroline**
- **Ceftazidime**
- **Ceftobiprole**
- **Ceftriaxone**
- **Cefuroxime**

Compound antibiotics

Some antibiotics are **co**mpounds (hence the prefix '**co**-') to augment their effectiveness. To give a few examples: co-amoxiclav combines amoxicillin (see section 'Penicillins') with clavulanic acid (a beta-lactamase inhibitor); co-fluampicil is a mixture of flucloxacillin and ampicillin; co-trimoxazole combines trimethoprim (see folic acid inhibitors) with sulfamethoxazole (see sulfonamide antibiotics); piperacillin is combined with tazobactam (a beta-lactamase inhibitor); ticarcillin can be given together with clavulanic acid.

- **Co-amoxiclav**
- **Co-fluampicil**
- **Co-trimoxazole**
- **Piperacillin with tazobactam**
- **Ticarcillin with clavulanic acid**

Folic acid inhibitors

Folic acid (vitamin B9) is essential for cell growth. Folic acid inhibitors work as 'bacteriostatic' agents (stopping bacteria from multiplying) by depriving bacteria of the folic acid that they need in order to reproduce (Barber and Robertson, 2015, p. 68). **Trime**tho**prim** can be given as monotherapy – on its own – or together with sulfameth**oxazole** (see sulfonamide antibiotics) to make the compound antibiotic **co-trimoxazole**, the two being 'bactericidal' (bacteria-killing) when given together.

- **Trimethoprim**

Lincosamides

Clindamycin is given to treat osteomyelitis, peritonitis, cellulitis or penicillin-resistant bacteria.

- **Clindamycin**

Lipopeptides and glycopeptides

The lipopeptide (daptomycin) and glycopeptide (dalbavancin, teicoplanin, telavancin and vancomycin) antibiotics are sometimes called 'antibiotics of last resort' and so tend to be reserved for the treatment of difficult-to-treat, antibiotic-resistant infections (Santos-Beneit et al., 2017). The letters '-**van**-' seen in most glycopeptide names derives from the word '**van**quish' and gives some indication of just how powerful and effective these antibacterial agents can be.

- **Dalbavancin**
- **Daptomycin**
- **Teicoplanin**
- **Telavancin**
- **Vancomycin**

Macrocyclic antibiotics

Fidaxomicin is the first in a new class of macrocyclic antibiotics (related to the macrolide antibiotics) that is used to treat *Clostridium difficile* ('C-diff') infection.

- **Fidaxomicin**

Macrolides

Macrolides are used to treat a variety of infections, including those of the respiratory tract and skin. Mac**ro**lide antibiotic names end in '-**thromycin**':

- **Azithromycin**

- **Clarithromycin**
- **Erythromycin**

Nitrofuran derivatives

Nitrofurantoin is given to treat urinary tract infections.

- **Nitrofurantoin**

Nitroimidazoles

The **nitroimidazole** class antibiotics are used to treat anaerobic bacterial infections, protozoa, leg ulcers and to help in the eradication of *Helicobacter pylori*.

- **Metronidazole**
- **Tinidazole**

Do not mistake **nitroimidazole** class antibiotics with names ending in '-**nidazole**' for other antibiotics with names ending in '-**oxazole**' (i.e., **sulfamethoxazole**: see sulfonamides); or for antifungal agents ending in '-**conazole**' (i.e., **fluconazole**); or for PPIs with names ending in '-**prazole**' (i.e., **lansoprazole**: see Chapter 1); or for hormone antagonists with names ending in '-**rozole**' (i.e., **anastrozole**: see Chapter 10) or for the azole-derivative antithyroid drug **carbimazole**.

Oxazolidinones

The oxa**zolid**inones are powerful antibiotics reserved for the treatment of drug-resistant bacteria, those commonly referred to as 'superbugs': methicillin-resistant *Staphylococcus aureus* (MRSA) and vancomycin-resistant *S. aureus* (VRSA).

- **Linezolid**
- **Tedizolid**

Penicillins

Penicillin is one of the earliest and remains the most well-known antibiotic. Its introduction in the 1940s transformed antimicrobial therapy. The peni**cillin**s are bactericidal and they work by undermining the integrity of the bacterial cell wall (Miele, 2017, pp. 163–164).

- **Amoxicillin**
- **Ampicillin**

- **Benzylpenicillin**
- **Flucloxacillin**
- **Phenoxymethylpenicillin**
- **Piperacillin (with tazobactam)**
- **Pivmecillinam**
- **Temocillin**
- **Ticarcillin (with clavulanic acid)**

Note: the rheumatoid arthritis drug **penicillamine** is not an antibiotic. However, its '**penicill-**' prefix is an indication that it was originally derived from **penicillin**.

Quinolones

Quinolones are broad-spectrum antibiotics used to treat a wide range of infections, including those of the urinary and respiratory tracts. Quinolone name stems have the distinctive looking suffix '-**floxacin**':

- **Ciprofloxacin**
- **Levofloxacin**
- **Moxifloxacin**
- **Ofloxacin**

Rifamycins

The prefix '**rifa-**' in rifamycin comes from the French slang word 'rififi', loosely translated as 'fight' or 'trouble' (the same linguistic origins as the English phrase 'riff-raff'). *Rififi* was the title of a famous 1950s French film and – surprising as it may seem – it was chosen as the prefix in rifamycin antibiotic names simply because the film *Rififi* was a favourite among those who were developing these bacteria-fighting drugs at the time (Aronson, 1999). Rifampicin is used to fight serious infections such as endocarditis and legionnaire's disease. Squire (2014, p. 88) explains that rifampicin has antimycobacterial properties, which means that it can also be used to treat mycobacterium-based infections such as tuberculosis (TB) and leprosy.

- **Rifabutin**
- **Rifampicin**
- **Rifaximin**

Sulfonamides

Sulfadiazine is used to prevent rheumatic fever recurrence. Sulfamethoxazole is given in combination with trimethoprim to create the compound antibiotic co-trimoxazole. Sulfonamides have generic names beginning with the prefix '**sulfa**-':

- **Sulfadiazine**
- **Sulfameth**oxazole

Despite its '**sulfa**-' prefix, do not mistake the aminosalicylate **sulfasalazine** (see Chapter 1) for a sulfonamide class antibacterial agent.

Tetracyclines and glycylcyclines

Tetracyclines have a broad spectrum of activity and can be used to treat MRSA, chlamydia and infections of the urinary tract. They work by inhibiting protein synthesis in bacteria (Török et al., 2009, p. 36). Tigecycline is a glycyl-cycline, the first in a new class of antibacterial agents closely related to the tetracyclines. Tetracycline and glycylcycline names end in '-**cycline**'.

- **Demeclo**cycline
- **Doxy**cycline
- **Lyme**cycline
- **Mino**cycline
- **Oxytetra**cycline
- **Tetra**cycline
- **Tige**cycline

Antifungals

Antifungals are given to treat fungal infections. Nystatin and amphotericin (the latter's '-**cin**' suffix indicating a link with macrolide class antibiotics) are polyene class antifungals; echinocandin class antifungals have names end-ing in '-**fungin**'; most imid**azole** and tri**azole** class antifungal names end in '-**conazole**'. The list below includes most of the antifungals in current use.

- **Amphoteric**in
- **Anidulafungin**
- **Caspofungin**

- Clotrimazole
- Econazole
- Fluconazole
- Isavuconazole
- Itraconazole
- Ketoconazole
- Micafungin
- Miconazole
- Nystatin
- Posaconazole
- Terbinafine
- Tioconazole
- Voriconazole

Do not confuse antifungal drugs ending in '-**conazole**' with antibacterials that end in either '-**oxazole**' (see sulfonamides) or '-**nidazole**' (see nitroimidazoles); or with PPIs ending in '-**prazole**' (i.e., ome**prazole**: see Chapter 1). Also, do not mistake **nystatin** for a cholesterol-lowering drug (see statins: Chapter 3).

Antivirals

Antivirals are drugs used to treat infection caused by a virus (as distinct from a bacterial or fungal infection). Antiviral drugs try to stop viruses from multiplying (different types doing so in different ways). Antivirals should be distinguished from vaccines. Vaccines are given in prophylaxis: to prevent viral infections from occurring; whereas antiviral agents are used to treat viral infections that have already taken hold.

Antiviral agents can include nucleoside analogues, nucleotide analogues, neuraminidase inhibitors, phosphonic acid derivatives, hepatitis C virus (HCV) inhibitors, protease inhibitors and interferons. Aciclovir is a nucleoside analogue and is perhaps the best-known of the antiviral drugs. It is used to treat herpes simplex (cold sores) and varicella-zoster (chicken pox) and works by interfering with viral DNA synthesis, stopping the virus from replicating itself (Gillespie and Bamford, 2012, p. 65). Some nucleoside analogues are used in the treatment of hepatitis B (i.e., entecavir) or hepatitis C (i.e., ribavirin). Oseltamivir and zanamivir are neuraminidase inhibitors given to treat influenza (neuraminidase being an enzyme that helps the influenza virus to multiply).

Interferons are immunostimulants that 'interfere' with viral replication: they are used to treat viral infections (hepatitis B and C), multiple sclerosis and certain types of cancer. HCV inhibitors (i.e., elbasvir) selectively target the hepatitis C virus. Protease inhibitors (i.e., grazoprevir) block the protease enzymes that facilitate viral proliferation. Two (sometimes three) different types of antiviral agent given together can be more potent and effective: for example, elbasvir (a HCV inhibitor) can be combined with grazoprevir (a hepatitis C-affecting protease inhibitor).

Most anti**vir**al drugs – regardless of type – have generic names that end in or contain the letters '-**vir**-': hepatitis C-affecting protease inhibitor drug names end in '-**previr**'; neur**ami**nidase inhibitors have names ending in '-**amivir**'; **fos**carnet sodium is a derivative of **phos**phonic acid. The prefix '**peg-**' in **peginterferon** comes from the word '**peg**ylated', meaning that it has undergone a process that prolongs the time that the drug is active in the bloodstream. In the summer of 2020 the antiviral agent **remdesivir** and **interferon** beta were being trialled as treatments for coronavirus disease 2019 (COVID-19). Listed below are just some of the many antivirals and interferons in current use:

- **Aciclovir**
- **Adefovir dipivoxil**
- **Elbasvir with grazoprevir**
- **Entecavir**
- **Famciclovir**
- **Foscarnet sodium**
- **Ganciclovir**
- **Interferon alfa**
- **Interferon beta**
- **Ledipasvir with sofosbuvir**
- **Oseltamivir**
- **Peginterferon alfa**
- **Remdesivir**
- **Ribavirin**
- **Valaciclovir**
- **Valganciclovir**
- **Zanamivir**

Antiretrovirals

Throughout history, humans have been subject to pandemics brought on by deadly infectious diseases (plague, smallpox, yellow fever, measles, tuberculosis, influenza, etc.). However, in the mid-to-late twentieth century, it seemed to many that, with antibiotics to treat bacterial infections and vaccines to prevent viral infections (together with modern public health services), the microbe had finally been brought under control. But in the early 1980s reports from the USA and sub-Saharan Africa about a new disease that could not be cured by any known medicine began to undermine confidence in science's ability to protect us all from life-threatening infectious diseases. Known as 'acquired immunodeficiency syndrome' (AIDS), it was found that this new disease was caused by a previously unknown retrovirus called the 'human immunodeficiency virus' (HIV). The battle against this deadly virus would push drug research into new directions and expand the boundaries of medicinal science. Antiretrovirals are drugs given to fight retroviruses. They include fusion (or entry) inhibitors, nucleoside (and non-nucleoside) reverse transcriptase inhibitors, protease inhibitors and integrase inhibitors; with different kinds of antiretroviral agent affecting different elements in the process by which HIV integrates itself into the DNA of cells in the human body. The first drug to treat AIDS (zidovudine) was approved for use in 1987. The protease inhibitors saquinavir and ritonavir were licenced for use in 1996, and within two years the mortality from AIDS was declining rapidly (Lichtenberg, 2003). While not a cure, antiretroviral agents are now slowing, or even halting, the progress of AIDS and turning it into a chronic, medically manageable condition.

Integrase inhibitor drug names end in '-**tegravir**'; the HIV-affecting protease inhibitors have names ending in '-**navir**'; other antiretro**vir**als end in '-**vudine**' or simply include the letters '-**vir**-' in their name. The list below incudes many (but not all) of the antiretrovirals in current use:

- **Abacavir**
- **Atazanavir**
- **Darunavir**
- **Dolutegravir**
- **Efavirenz**
- **Elvitegravir**
- **Enfuvirtide**
- **Etravirine**
- **Fosamprenavir**
- **Lamivudine**
- **Maraviroc**
- **Nevirapine**
- **Raltegravir**
- **Rilpivirine**

- Ritonavir
- Saquinavir
- Stavudine
- Tenofovir disoproxil
- Tipranavir
- Zidovudine

References

Aronson, J. (1999). That's show business. *British Medical Journal*, 319 (7215), 972.

Barber, P. and Robertson, D. (2015). *Essentials of pharmacology for nurses*. 3rd ed. Maidenhead: Open University Press.

Gillespie, S. and Bamford, K. (2012). *Medical microbiology and infection at a glance*. 4th ed. Chichester: Wiley Blackwell.

Lichtenberg, F.R. (2003). The effect of new drug approvals on HIV mortality in the USA, 1987–1998. *Economics and Human Biology*, 1 (2), 259–266 [online]. Available from: doi: 10.1016/S1570-677X(02)00031-X.

Miele, M.B. (2017). Principles of antimicrobial action and resistance. In: Tille, P.M. (ed). *Bailey and Scott's diagnostic microbiology*. 14th ed. St. Louis: Elsevier, pp. 161–176.

Santos-Beneit, F., Ordóñez-Robles, M. and Martin, J.A. (2017). Glycopeptide resistance: links with inorganic phosphate metabolism and cell envelope stress. *Biochemical Pharmacology* [online]. Available from: doi: 10.1016/j.bcp.2016.11.017.

Squire, B. (2014). Tuberculosis. In: Beeching, N. and Gill, G. (eds). *Tropical medicine lecture notes*. 7th ed. Chichester: Wiley Blackwell, pp. 82–95.

Török, E., Moran, E. and Cooke, F. (2009). *Oxford handbook of infectious diseases and microbiology*. Oxford: Oxford University Press.

Alkylating agents
Antimetabolites
Cytotoxic antibiotics
Platinum compounds
Proteasome inhibitors
Protein kinase inhibitors
Tyrosine kinase inhibitors
Taxanes
Topoisomerase inhibiting agents
Vinca alkaloids
Sex hormones and hormone antagonists
Analogues of thalidomide
Antiproliferative immunosuppressants
Calcineurin inhibitors and 'non-calcineurin' inhibitors
Monoclonal antibodies

Chemotherapy

Chemotherapy agents are used to treat neoplastic disorders (cancer). Chemotherapy drugs try to stop cancer from spreading by interfering with the way that cancer cells divide and replicate. In addition to the main chemotherapy agents listed on the pages that follow, note that sex hormones and hormone antagonists, immunomodulating agents, interferons (see Chapter 9) and corticosteroids (see Chapter 8) can also play a role in the treatment of cancer.

The Drug Recognition Guide, Second Edition. Mark Currivan.
© 2021 John Wiley & Sons Ltd. Published 2021 by John Wiley & Sons Ltd.

Alkylating agents

The first alkylating chemotherapy medicines were derived from the chemical warfare agent **must**ard gas (Smith, 2017). Alkylating agents damage cancer cell DNA, affecting its ability to divide. Suffixes seen among the alkylating agents include '-**mustine**' (indicating a nitrogen **must**ard derivative), '-**phosphamide**' (and its homophone '-**fosfamide**') and '-**sulfan**':

- **Benda**mustine**
- **Bu**sulfan**
- **Carmustine**
- **Chlorambucil**
- **Cyclophosphamide**
- **Estramustine**
- **Ifosfamide**
- **Lomustine**
- **Melphalan**
- **Temozolomide**
- **Thiotepa**
- **Treo**sulfan**

Antimetabolites

'Antimetabolite' is a broad term applied to a diverse group of medicines that work by interfering with cancer cell metabolism, inhibiting folate-dependent enzymes and so inducing cancer cell death. Methotrexate – the most well-known antimetabolite – is an antifolate (folic acid antagonist) prescribed for its antineoplastic and anti-inflammatory properties (O'Shaughnessy, 2018, pp. 306–307). Note that pentostatin (see section 'Cytotoxic antibiotics') could also be classified as an antimetabolite. Most antimetabolites have names ending in '-**arabine**', '-**citabine**', '-**trexed**' or '-**trexate**'.

- **Azacitidine**
- **Cape**citabine**
- **Cladribine**
- **Clof**arabine**
- **Cyt**arabine**
- **Decitabine**
- **Flud**arabine**
- **Fluorouracil**
- **Gemcitabine**
- **Mercaptopurine**

- **Metho**trexate
- **Nel**arabine
- **Peme**trexed
- **Ralti**trexed

 Despite ending in '-**tidine**', do not mistake **azacitidine** for a H2-receptor antagonist (see Chapter 1).

Cytotoxic antibiotics

The cytotoxic antibiotics (including the anthracyclines) should not be mistaken for antibacterial agents (see Chapter 9), instead their extreme toxicity makes the cytotoxic antibiotics suitable only for use as drugs to intentionally damage rapidly dividing cancer cells.

- **Bleomycin**
- **Daunorubicin**
- **Doxorubicin**
- **Epirubicin**
- **Idarubicin**
- **Mitomycin**
- **Mitoxantrone**
- **Pentostatin**
- **Pixantrone**

 Despite ending in '-**statin**', do not mistake **pentostatin** for a cholesterol-lowering drug (see statins: Chapter 3).

Platinum compounds

Platinum-based compounds work as anticancer agents by damaging cancer cell DNA. Cisplatin was the first **platin**um compound and, despite its potential nephrotoxicity (Crona et al., 2017), it remains one of the most potent and effective anticancer drugs.

- **Carboplatin**
- **Cisplatin**
- **Oxaliplatin**

Proteasome inhibitors

Proteasome helps break down and degrade protein. Drugs that inhibit the action of proteasome are used in the treatment of multiple myeloma. Proteasome inhibitors have names ending in '-**zomib**':

- **Bortezomib**
- **Carfilzomib**
- **Ixazomib**

Protein (and tyrosine) kinase inhibitors

Protein kinases are enzymes that help regulate cell activity; consequently, drugs that inhibit these enzymes target their effects on rapidly dividing cancer cells. Many protein kinase inhibitors (PKIs) are specific tyrosine kinase inhibitors (TKIs) used in 'targeted' chemotherapy. Below are just a few of the growing number of PKIs and TKIs in current use:

- **Dasatinib**
- **Erlotinib**
- **Everolimus**
- **Gefitinib**
- **Ibrutinib**
- **Imatinib**
- **Lapatinib**
- **Nilotinib**
- **Pazopanib**
- **Temsirolimus**

Taxanes

The bark of the **Pac**ific yew tree (or **tax**us brevifolia) contains a toxin called **tax**ane that was used to develop the cancer-fighting medicines that bear the same name (Neal, 2016, p. 89). Taxane names end in '-**taxel**':

- **Cabazitaxel**
- **Docetaxel**
- **Paclitaxel**

Topoisomerase-inhibiting agents

The enzymes topoisomerase I and II help regulate DNA. Inhibiting these enzymes interferes with the DNA in rapidly changing cancer cells, causing the DNA to unwind. Derived from natural chemicals extracted from the camptotheca acuminata tree, irinotecan and **topotecan** inhibit **topo**isomerase I. Etoposide is a podophyllotoxin derivative: a medicine based on toxins extracted from the podophyllum plant (the American mandrake or mayapple). Podophyllotoxins have a toxic effect on **topo**isomerase II enzymes and so are used in the anticancer drug e**topo**side. **Topo**isomerase-inhibiting agents have generic names that feature the letters '-**topo**-' or the suffix '-**tecan**', sometimes both:

- **Etoposide**
- **Irinotecan**
- **Topotecan**

Do not mistake the antiepileptic drug **topiramate** (see Chapter 5) for a **topo**isomerase-inhibiting agent.

Vinca alkaloids

It is estimated that about a quarter of all modern medicines have their origins in chemicals obtained from plants from various parts of the world, for example: anti-inflammatory drugs from willow (see aminosalicylates); digoxin from the fox-glove (see cardiac glycosides); atropine from *Atropa belladonna* (see antimus-carinics); paclitaxel from the Pacific yew tree (see taxanes). On the Indian Ocean island of Madagascar, there is a flowering plant called the *Catharanthus roseus*, formerly known as the **vin**ca rosea. Colloquially referred to as the 'Madagascan periwinkle', people native to the island have been using extracts from this plant in herbal remedies for centuries. The modern medicines known as **vin**ca alka-loids were originally derived from chemicals extracted from the *C. roseus* (McFadden, 2013, pp. 303–304). Like many medicinal plants, the *C. roseus* is poisonous; however, when its active ingredient is given in a carefully calibrated dose, it is selectively toxic to cancer cells. The cytotoxic action of the vinca alka-loids is due to their effect on cell microtubule function. Without effectively func-tioning microtubules, cells cannot divide; and if cancer cells cannot divide, they cannot multiply and spread. Vinca alkaloids are given to treat leukaemia, lym-phoma and some cancers of the breast and lung.

- **Vinblastine**
- **Vincristine**
- **Vindesine**
- **Vinflunine**
- **Vinorelbine**

Sex hormones and hormone antagonists

Some hormone-responsive cancers (i.e., breast cancer in women or prostate cancer in men) grow more rapidly in the presence of sex hormone activity. The properties of sex hormones and hormone antagonists can be used to slow down or stop the growth of hormone-responsive cancers (also see section 'Chemotherapy'). Sex hormones and hormone antagonists are also used in the treatment of urinary obstruction, endometriosis, contraception and infertility.

Antioestrogens block oestrogen receptors and are used to treat oestrogen-receptor-positive tumours such as breast cancer. Aromatase inhibitors deprive breast cancer cells of the oestrogen they utilise to grow and spread. The oestrogen ethinylestradiol and the progestogen norethisterone (hormones commonly given together in the combined contraceptive pill) can be prescribed separately in cancer therapy, with ethinylestradiol used palliatively in prostate cancer and norethisterone given in breast cancer. Antiandrogens are used to treat hormone-responsive cancer or a benign enlargement of the prostate. The enzyme 5α-reductase is involved in the metabolism of testosterone and so 5α-reductase inhibitors are a particular type of antiandrogen that is used to relieve urinary obstruction in men with benign prostatic hyperplasia (BPH) and which work by causing an enlarged prostate to regress (shrink), thereby improving urine outflow in situations where the passage of urine has been obstructed by prostatic enlargement.

Gonadotropin-releasing hormones are used to treat breast cancer, prostate cancer and endometriosis. Anti-gonadotropin-releasing hormones are used in prostate cancer and infertility treatment.

Antio**estr**ogen drug names end in the letters '-**estr**ant', '-**oxifen**' or '-**ifene**'; aromatase inhibitors have names ending in either '-**est**ane' or '-**rozole**'; antiandrogens end in '-**lutamide**' or '-**ter**one'; 5α-reductase inhibitor drug names end in '-**steride**' (5α-reductase is an enzyme involved in testo**ster**one metabolism); gonadotropin-releasing hormone names end in '-**relin**'; while anti-gonadotropin-releasing hormone names end in '-**relix**':

- **Abira**ter**one**
- **Anastrozole**
- **Apa**lutamide
- **Bica**lutamide
- **Buserelin**
- **Degarelix**
- **Duta**ster**ide**
- **Enza**lutamide

- **Ethinylestradiol**
- **Exemestane**
- **Finasteride**
- **Flutamide**
- **Fulvestrant**
- **Goserelin**
- **Letrozole**
- **Leuprorelin**
- **Norethisterone**
- **Tamoxifen**
- **Toremifene**
- **Triptorelin**

Immunomodulating agents

Immunomodulating agents suppress or modifies the way that the body's immune system works. They are used in the treatment of autoimmune disorders, chronic inflammatory conditions, to help prevent the rejection of a transplanted organ, or as part of cancer therapy. Also see sections 'Chemotherapy' and 'Corticosteroids' (see Chapter 8).

Analogues of thalidomide

Thalidomide and its analogues are immunomodulating medicines with angiogenesis-inhibiting properties that are now being used to treat cancer. Thalidomide was initially developed as a sedative. It was found that it worked as an antiemetic and in the late 1950s and early 1960s it was given to pregnant women as a treatment for morning sickness. But serious birth defects were found in babies born to women who had taken the drug and it was eventually withdrawn (the notorious 'thalidomide babies' scandal). Decades later, however, the drug began to be re-evaluated. It was realised that the very side effect that had made the drug so dangerous to a baby developing in the womb – inhibiting the growth of new blood vessels (inhibition of angiogenesis) – meant that it could be used as an anticancer treatment (Airley, 2009, pp. 209–212). Analogues of thalidomide (with angiogenesis-inhibition as a mechanism of action) deprive cancer cells of the microscopic blood supply they require in order to develop and spread.

- **Lenalidomide**
- **Pomalidomide**
- **Thalidomide**

Antiproliferative immunosuppressants

When organ transplantation takes place, the recipient's body produces a proliferation of lymphocytes (white blood cells) that – unhelpfully – try to reject this 'foreign' tissue. Antiproliferative drugs are given to block this proliferation of lymphocytes, thereby suppressing organ transplant rejection. Azathioprine could also be classified as an antimetabolite (see antimetabolites).

- **Azathioprine**
- **Mycophenolate mofetil**

Calcineurin and 'non-calcineurin' inhibiting immunosuppressants

T-cells (a type of white blood cell) play a key role in the immune system. They are activated by an enzyme called calcineurin. Calcineurin inhibitors exert their immunosuppressive effects by blocking calcineurin. Sirol**imus** is called a 'non-calcineurin-inhibiting immunosuppressant' because, while its effects are like those of tacrol**imus**, its action is not directly related to calcineurin inhibition (the drug's **imunos**uppressant properties being illustrated by its '-**imus**' name stem). Note that eve**rolimus** and temsi**rolimus** (see section 'Protein kinase inhibitors') are both derivatives of si**rolimus** (hence the same '-**rolimus**' suffix).

- **Ciclosporin**
- **Pimecrolimus**
- **Sirolimus**
- **Tacrolimus**

Monoclonal antibodies

Monoclonal antibodies are synthetic antibodies designed to bind to proteins on the surface of targeted cells in order to stimulate the person's immune system to identify and attack those particular cells. This precise targeting means that monoclonal antibodies can be used to treat a wide variety of cancers, autoimmune disorders (i.e., ANCA-associated vasculitis) and an increasing number of other conditions (Shah et al., 2012). Some monoclonal antibodies are now being used to lower cholesterol (see Chapter 3), some to treat respiratory disorders (see Chapter 4), some for rheumatoid arthritis or Crohn's (i.e., adalimumab and infliximab), or multiple sclerosis (i.e., natalizumab), or migraine (i.e., erenumab). **M**onoclonal **anti**bodies – just a few representative examples of which are listed below – have generic names ending in '-**mab**':

- **Adalimumab**
- **Bevacizumab**

- Cetuximab
- Erenumab
- Infliximab
- Natalizumab
- Olaratumab
- Panitumumab
- Pertuzumab
- Rituximab
- Siltuximab
- Trastuzumab

References

Airley, R. (2009). *Cancer chemotherapy*. Chichester: Wiley Blackwell.

Crona, D.J., Faso, A., Nishijima, T.F. et al. (2017). A systematic review of strategies to prevent cisplatin-induced nephrotoxicity. *The Oncologist*, 22 (5), 609–619 [online]. Wiley Online Library. Available from: doi: 10.1634/theoncologist.2016-0319.

McFadden, R. (2013). *Introducing pharmacology: for nursing and healthcare*. 2nd ed. London: Routledge.

Neal, M.J. (2016). *Medical pharmacology at a glance*. 8th ed. Chichester: Wiley.

O'Shaughnessy, K.M. (ed.) (2018). *British Medical Association concise guide to medication and drugs*. 6th ed. London: Dorling Kindersley.

Shah, Y., Mohiuddin, A., Sluman, C. et al. (2012). Rituximab in anti-glomerular basement membrane disease. *Quarterly Journal of Medicine: International Journal of Medicine*, 105 (2), 195–197.

Smith, S.L. (2017). War! What is it good for? Mustard gas medicine. *Canadian Medical Association Journal*, 189 (8), E321–E322 [online]. Available from: doi: 10.1503/cmaj.161032.

Index of Drug Groups

The Drug Recognition Guide, Second Edition. Mark Currivan.
© 2021 John Wiley & Sons Ltd. Published 2021 by John Wiley & Sons Ltd.

Index of Drugs

The Drug Recognition Guide, Second Edition. Mark Currivan.
© 2021 John Wiley & Sons Ltd. Published 2021 by John Wiley & Sons Ltd.